Skin Diseases of the Cat

Other titles of interest

Skin Diseases of the Dog
Sue Paterson
0 632 04808 5

Canine Medicine and Therapeutics
Fourth edition
Edited by Neil T. Gorman
0 632 04045 9

Allen's Fertility and Obstetrics in the Dog
Second edition
Gary C. W. England
0 632 04806 9

Cardiorespiratory Diseases of the Dog and Cat
M. Martin and B. Corcoran
0 632 03298 7

Canine and Feline Geriatrics
M. Davies
0 632 03479 3

Diseases of Domestic Guinea Pigs
V. C. G. Richardson
0 632 03301 0

Diseases of Small Domestic Rodents
V. C. G. Richardson
0 632 04132 3

Diseases of Domestic Rabbits
Second edition
L. Okerman
0 632 03804 7

Diagnostic Ultrasound in the Dog and Cat
Frances Barr
0 632 02845 9

Skin Diseases of the Cat

Sue Paterson, MA, VetMB, DVD, DipECVD, MRCVS

Veterinary Dermatology Service
Animal Medical Centre
Chorlton
Manchester

Blackwell
Science

© 2000 by
Blackwell Science Ltd
Editorial Offices:
Osney Mead, Oxford OX2 0EL
25 John Street, London WC1N 2BL
23 Ainslie Place, Edinburgh EH3 6AJ
350 Main Street, Malden
  MA 02148 5018, USA
54 University Street, Carlton
  Victoria 3053, Australia
10, rue Casimir Delavigne
  75006 Paris, France

Other Editorial Offices:

Blackwell Wissenschafts-Verlag GmbH
Kurfürstendamm 57
10707 Berlin, Germany

Blackwell Science KK
MG Kodenmacho Building
7-10 Kodenmacho Nihombashi
Chuo-ku, Tokyo 104, Japan

First published 2000

Set in 10/12 pt Palatino
by Best-set Typesetter Ltd., Hong Kong
Printed and bound in Spain by
Hostench, Barcelona

The Blackwell Science logo is a
trade mark of Blackwell Science Ltd,
registered at the United Kingdom
Trade Marks Registry

DISTRIBUTORS

Marston Book Services Ltd
PO Box 269
Abingdon
Oxon OX14 4YN
(*Orders*: Tel: 01235 465500
            Fax: 01235 465555)

USA
Blackwell Science, Inc.
Commerce Place
350 Main Street
Malden, MA 02148 5018
(*Orders*: Tel: 800 759 6102
                  781 388 8250
            Fax: 781 388 8255)

Canada
Login Brothers Book Company
324 Saulteaux Crescent
Winnipeg, Manitoba R3J 3T2
(*Orders*: Tel: 204 837 2987
            Fax: 204 837 3116)

Australia
Blackwell Science Pty Ltd
54 University Street
Carlton, Victoria 3053
(*Orders*: Tel: 03 9347 0300
            Fax: 03 9347 5001)

A catalogue record for this title
is available from the British Library

ISBN 0-632-04805-0

Library of Congress
Cataloging-in-Publication Data
is available

For further information on
Blackwell Science, visit our website:
www.blackwell-science.com

To Richard, Samantha, Matthew and Mum and Dad.
For their love and support

Acknowledgements

To all the friends and colleagues in practice who have helped,
encouraged and inspired me throughout my dermatological career.

Contents

Abbreviations

ACTH	Adrenocorticotrophic hormone
ALT	Alanine aminotransferase
ANA	Antinuclear antibody
AST	Aspartate transaminase
CT	Computer tomography
DTM	Dermatophyte test medium
ECG	Electrocardiogram
FHV	Feline herpes virus
FeLV	Feline leukaemia virus
FeSV	Feline sarcoma virus
FIP	Feline infectious peritonitis
FIV	Feline immunodeficiency virus
FT_3	Free triiodothyronine
FT_4	Free thyroxine
IGF-1	Insulin-like growth factor-1
LDH	Lactate dehydrogenase
MRI	Magnetic resonance imaging
OCD	Obsessive-compulsive disorder
PPA	Pancreatic paraneoplastic alopecia
SAP	Serum alkaline phosphatase
TRH	Thyrotropin releasing hormone
TSH	Thyroid stimulating hormone
TT_3	Total triiodothyronine
TT_4	Total thyroxine
UV	Ultraviolet

Chapter 1

Introduction

Feline skin disease forms an integral and important part of feline medicine. The cat is now recognised as a distinct and unique species; it responds in many different ways to a whole range of pathogens. Previous texts have aimed to group the cat and dog together dermatologically. However fungal, viral and bacterial pathogens affect the feline skin in a different way to the canine counterpart. A common misconception is that alopecia in the cat is often endocrine in origin: we now know that most alopecia in this species is usually traumatic and rarely due to systemic disease. Despite the differences in the disease presentations feline skin shares many structural and functional similarities with the dog.

Basic functions include:

- Prevents loss of water, electrolytes and macromolecules.
- Mechanical protection.
- Provides elasticity to allow movement.
- Nerve sensors allow perception of heat, cold, pressure, pain and itching.
- Temperature regulation.
- Storage of vitamins, electrolytes, water, fat, carbohydrates and protein.
- Immune regulation to prevent development of infection and neoplasia.
- Antibacterial and antifungal activity.
- Vitamin D production.
- Pigment production to protect against solar damage.

STRUCTURE OF THE SKIN

Epidermis

- Most superficial layer of the skin composed of:
  - Keratinocytes ~85%.
  - Langerhans cells ~5–8%.
  - Melanocytes ~5%.

Keratinocytes

- Produce structural keratins.
- Phagocytic – capable of processing antigens.
- Produce cytokines to stimulate or inhibit the immune response.

Langerhans cells

- Suprabasilar dendritic cells.
- Important epidermal antigen presenting cells.
- Phagocytic – capable of processing antigens.
- Able to migrate to lymphatics to present antigen to antigen specific T cells.

Melanocytes

- Dendritic cells – their cytoplastic extensions (dendrites) communicate with 10–20 keratinocytes to form an 'epidermal melanin unit'.
- Produce eumelanin or pheomelanin within melanosomes through series of steps from tyrosine.
- Melanosomes containing pigment migrate to the end of dendrites and transfer melanin to adjacent epidermal cells.

Epidermal structure

- Stratum basale.
- Stratum spinosum.
- Stratum granulosum.
- Stratum lucidum.
- Stratum corneum.

Stratum basale

- Columnar cells, tightly adherent to the basement membrane.
- Site of initial keratin production.

Stratum spinosum

- Cells polyhedral, becoming flattened.
- This layer is particularly thick in footpads, nasal planum and at mucocutaneous junctions.
- Keratin production accelerates and is formed into bundles.
- Lamellar granule synthesis starts.

Stratum granulosum

- Flattened cells.
- Keratohyline granules visible rich in profilaggrin.
- Profilaggrin converted to filaggrin, which acts to bind keratin filaments.
- Lamellar granules discharge into intercellular space to form lipid rich lamellae between cells.
- Degeneration of cell organelles and nucleus.

Stratum lucidum

- Compact layer of dead keratinocytes found only in footpads and nasal planum.

Stratum corneum

- Flattened cornified cells constantly shed to balance the proliferation of basal cells.
- Transit time from stratum basale to stratum corneum ~22 days.
- Internal scaffold of keratin/filaggrin.
- External lipid rich cornified cell envelope.

Basement membrane zone

- This is the area that separates the epidermis from the dermis.
- Moving from the epidermis to the dermis it can be divided into:
  - Basal cell plasma membrane – contains the anchoring hemidesmosomes of basal cells.
  - Lamina lucida.
  - Lamina densa.
  - Sublamina densa – contains anchoring fibrils.

Dermis

- Fibres.
- Ground substance.
- Cells.
- Epidermal appendages.

Fibres

- Produced by fibroblasts.
- Collagenous (collagen) 80%.
  - Thick bands of multiple protein fibrils.
  - Provide tensile strength and some elasticity.
- Reticular.
  - Fine branching network of fibres.
- Elastin 4%.
  - Single fine branching structures bordering collagen bundles.
  - Provide elasticity.

Ground substance

- Produced by fibroblasts.
- Composed of glycosaminoglycans linked to proteoglycans.

- Provides dermal support, contributes to water storage, lubrication, growth and development.

Cells

- Fibroblasts.
- Melanocytes.
- Mast cells.

Epidermal appendages

Arrector pili muscle

- Smooth muscle originates in superficial dermis and inserts at bulge region of primary hair follicle.
- Contraction of muscle raises the hair (piloerection).
- Under cholinergic nerve control, piloerection associated with 'flight or fight'.
- Associated with thermoregulation, and emptying sebaceous glands.

Blood vessels

- Three intercommunicating plexuses of arteries and veins.
  - ○ Deep plexus – supplies subcutis, lower portions of hair follicle and epitrichial sweat gland.
  - ○ Middle plexus – supplies arrector pili muscle, middle portion of hair follicle and sebaceous gland.
  - ○ Superficial plexus – supplies upper portion of hair follicles and sends capillary loops up to the epidermis.
- Arteriovenous anastomoses.
  - ○ Connections between arteries and veins found especially in the deep dermis that allows blood to bypass the capillary bed.
  - ○ Most commonly seen in the extremities.

Lymph vessels

- Arise from capillary networks in superficial dermis and surround adnexal structures.

Nerves

- Sensory nerves.
  - ○ Subepidermal and intraepidermal plexus.
  - ○ Cutaneous endorgans within the dermis, e.g. tylotrich pad.
  - ○ Network around the hair follicle.
- Motor nerves.
  - ○ Arrector pili muscle.
  - ○ Epitrichial sweat gland.

Hair follicle

- Divided into three sections.
  - ○ Infundibulum – entrance of sebaceous gland to epithelial surface.
  - ○ Isthmus – entrance of sebaceous gland to attachment of arrector pili muscle.
  - ○ Inferior segment – attachment of arrector pili muscle to the dermal papilla.
- Compound hair follicle composed of a single large hair surrounded by up to five secondary hairs, emerging from a single hole.
- Each primary hair has:
  - ○ Arrector pili muscle.
  - ○ Sebaceous gland.
  - ○ Sweat gland (epitrichial).
- Each secondary hair usually has a sebaceous gland only.

Arrector pili muscle

- See epidermal appendages.

Sebaceous gland

- Distributed throughout haired skin – not found in footpad or nasal planum.
- Open through duct into hair follicle canal in the infundibular region.
- Large and numerous in sparsely haired areas especially mucocutaneous junctions and interdigital spaces. Also dorsal neck and rump.
- Oily sebum secretion thought to be under hormonal control.
  - ○ Physical barrier by lubrication and hydration of skin and hairs.
  - ○ Chemical barrier – sebum/sweat emulsion has antimicrobial activities.
  - ○ Pheromonal properties.

Sweat gland

Epitrichial (apocrine)

- Distributed throughout haired skin – not found in footpad or nasal planum.
- Localised below sebaceous glands, open through duct into hair follicle canal in the infundibular region above sebaceous gland opening.
- Large and numerous in sparsely haired areas as sebaceous glands.
- Rich blood supply to gland but not innervated; control thought to be by diffusion of neurotransmitters from the circulation.
- Secretion – apocrine sweat.
  - ○ Chemical barrier – secretion especially rich in IgA.
  - ○ Pheromonal properties.

Atrichial (eccrine)

- Found only in footpads not associated with hairs.
- Rich nerve supply; direct nerve control thought to occur.

Structure of hair follicle

- Dermal papilla.
- Hair matrix.
- Hair.
- Inner root sheath.
- Outer root sheath.

Dermal hair papilla

- Extension of dermal connective tissue covered by basement membrane.

Hair matrix

- Nucleated epithelial cells covering the papilla give rise to the hair and inner root sheath.

Hair

- Medulla – innermost region composed of longitudinal rows of cuboidal cells.
- Cortex – cornified spindle shaped cells, contain pigment to colour the hair.
- Cuticle – outermost layer of flattened cornified anuclear cells, form tiles that interlock with the cuticle of the inner root sheath.

Inner root sheath (IRS)

- Function of sheath is to mould the hair within it.
- Composed of three layers, all of which contain trichohyalin granules.
  ○ Innermost layer – inner root sheath cuticle is a single layer of overlapping cells.
  ○ Middle layer – Huxley's layer is 1–3 nucleated cell layers.
  ○ Outermost layer – Henle's layer is a layer of anuclear cells.

Outer root sheath (ORS)

- Downward extension of epidermis.
- In the infundibulum – keratinisation occurs with formation of keratohyline granules as in the rest of the epidermis.
- In the isthmus – tricholemmal keratinisation occurs.
- Below the level of the isthmus – no keratinisation occurs as ORS is covered by IRS.
- ORS is surrounded by:
  ○ Basement membrane/glassy membrane – downward extension of the epidermal basement membrane.
  ○ Fibrous root sheath – connective tissue layer.

The hair cycle

Anagen – growing phase

- New hair bulb forms – germ cells at base of follicle extend down to surround dermal papilla deep in the dermis.
- Well-developed dermal papilla covered by hair matrix identified. Matrix cells show mitotic activity ('ball and claw' appearance).

Catagen – intermediate phase

- Hair growth stops, papilla moves away from matrix cells as hair moves up in dermis.

Telogen – resting phase

- Dermal papilla separates from the bulb of matrix cells ('club' hair appearance).
- Pigment lost from bulb, no mitotic activity.

APPROACH TO THE FELINE CASE

Sceptics would group cat skin diseases into steroid responsive and steroid unresponsive problems. Unfortunately, because the cat is recognised as being a highly steroid tolerant species, this has led in the past to the overzealous use of potent glucocorticoids and progestagens, often administered at the insistence of the owners for a 'quick fix'. Increased owner awareness of the side effects of drugs has led to more recent trends to investigate feline skin problems rather than prescribe symptomatically. Clinicians offering expertise in both feline medicine and dermatology are more than happy to offer advice and referral for busy veterinary surgeons. However, as most small animal practitioners can expect 10–20% of their feline patients to present with skin problems, they should have some basic grounding in dermatology, even if this knowledge serves to distinguish the straightforward from the 'needs referral' cases.

History taking

Time is always the most important limiting factor when taking a history from a client. Often it is impossible to assess a patient during a normal consultation, and it is tempting to prescribe a symptomatic treatment during a busy clinic. This is a justifiable practice, providing the therapy that is supplied does not compromise the ability to investigate the problem more thoroughly at a later date. Antibiotics, antihistamines and topical therapy in the form of shampoos will rarely complicate a diagnosis. The response of a patient to such treatments can often help in directing further tests. Symptomatic steroid therapy is rarely indicated and often makes further investigations impossible in the short term.

History taking needs to be logical, and different clinicians approach their questioning in a different manner. Often the emphasis will be changed depending on the initial owner complaint.

History forms are used extensively by some clinicians, but the author does not use a preprinted sheet as she feels this tends not to encourage relevant questioning that can be varied for each case. The history itself can be divided into six sections.

Owner complaint

Cats are very secretive animals, and even the best history taken from the owner can be misleading. Cats will groom in private and often have a second 'home' where they are fed, groomed or medicated without the knowledge of your client. A history should always be interpreted in the light of clinical findings. Hair loss in the cat is usually of a traumatic origin; systemic disorders usually present with some overt signs of ill health other than just cutaneous lesions.

General details

The age, sex, breed, colour and weight of the animal can give important clues to the nature of the disease. For example, dermatophytosis is most commonly identified in young kittens.

General health

- Activity – over active, difficult to handle, e.g. hyperthyroidism.
- Appetite/thirst – increased in hyperadrenocorticism but also in steroid administration.
- Feeding – is the cat being fed a well balanced diet? The taurine, protein and essential acid levels are particularly important. Are large amounts of oily fish or liver being fed?
- Gastrointestinal signs – allergic bowel disease can occur concurrently with atopy. A history of hairballs suggests overgrooming.
- Urogenital signs – cystitis associated with hyperadrenocorticism, excessive progestagen administration. Cats may traumatise perineal area in association with urolithiasis.
- Cardiothoracic signs – tachycardia often seen in hyperthyroidism. Dyspnoea can occur with a thoracic mass such as a thymoma.
- Central nervous system signs – fits may occur in hyperadrenocorticism.
- Locomotor system signs – inability to jump with pansteatitis.
- Eye disease – conjunctivitis and keratitis can be seen in conjunction with viral diseases.
- Ear disease – ectopic *Otodectes* infestations can cause facial and perianal pruritus. Typical ear signs will be seen.
- Weight loss – associated with leukaemia virus, diabetes, hyperthyroidism.

Environmental history

- Other in contact animals, either pets or wild animals. Small rodents may act as a source of dermatophytes; rabbits may transmit *Cheyletiella*.

- Human contacts, signs of owner contagion especially ringworm, *Cheyletiella* (Fig. 1.1).
- Animal's environment – does the cat live indoors or outdoors? Is it in a rural environment? Does the cat hunt? Bite wounds may be an initial source of pox virus infection (Fig. 1.2).

Dermatological history

- When did the symptoms first appear?
- What part of the body was first affected?
- Progression of the disease.

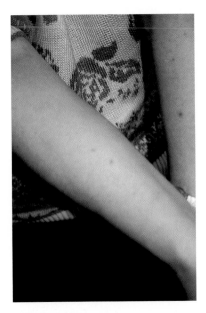

Fig. 1.1 Papular lesions of *Cheyletiella* on the arms of an owner.

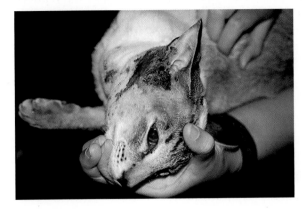

Fig. 1.2 Lesions of cat pox in a Siamese cat.

○ Has there ever been a seasonal pattern?
○ Pruritus? This can be difficult to assess in a cat (see section on trichography later in this chapter).

Previous therapy

- What is the cat like to medicate? Will it take tablets? Have unrealistic expectations been made of the owner to treat the cat?
- What previous therapy has been given and how has the cat responded to it?
- Flea treatment – what was used last, when was it last used and was it applied properly?

Examination of the animal

Once a history has been taken the animal can be examined. A general physical inspection should be undertaken in every case. A more detailed examination of some organ systems can be undertaken where indicated. Ophthalmological, neuromuscular examination including cranial nerve reflexes may be indicated in some systemic diseases.

Physical examination

- It is important to have adequate space, good owner and pet co-operation (sedation of fractious or nervous animals may be necessary), and good lighting.
- Before even touching the cat it is important to assess the animal's general appearance, demeanour, body condition.
- Temperature, pulse and respiratory rate should be checked.
- Mouth – especially the palate – a common site for eosinophilic granulomas (Fig. 1.3). Look for abnormalities of colour, e.g. jaundice (Fig. 1.4) and petechiation.

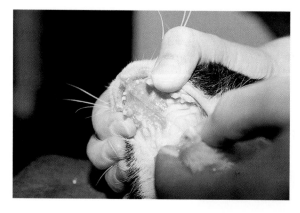

Fig. 1.3 Eosinophilic granuloma on the soft palate.

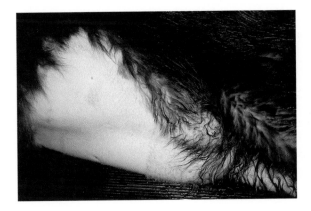

Fig. 1.4 Jaundice of ventral abdominal skin in a cat with FIP.

- Ears/eyes – are often affected as an extension of the skin disease. Cats are particularly prone to viral ocular disease, which should be differentiated from periocular skin disease.
- Palpation of peripheral lymph nodes – checking for localised or generalised lymphadenopathy which can be seen with neoplastic disease, bacterial or fungal infections.
- Auscultation of the chest – especially tachycardia seen with hyperthyroidism.
- Palpation of the abdomen – checking for abdominal masses; hepatomegaly may be seen with hyperadrenocorticism.
- Assessment of muscle development – pot bellied appearance with hyperadrenocorticism.

Dermatological examination

- This should include the whole of the skin and all of the mucous membranes.
- Has the cat given you any dermatological clues whilst it has been in the room?
- Is the cat sitting grooming during the consultation?

General assessment of the coat

- Seborrhoea – dry or greasy.
- Hair colour/texture – is the coat faded, have primary hairs been lost?
- Distribution of lesions – are these confined to particular areas or is the whole body involved?

Skin

- Don't just check the accessible areas of the skin, always turn the animal over to check the ventral abdominal skin and perineal areas (Fig. 1.5), as well as inside the mouth and ears; the perianal skin; interdigital spaces and footpads.
- Check the skin quality – atrophic/inelastic with hyperadrenocorticism, skin fragility syndrome.

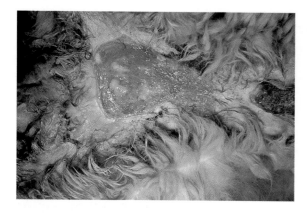

Fig. 1.5 Epidermal slough due to urethral rupture.

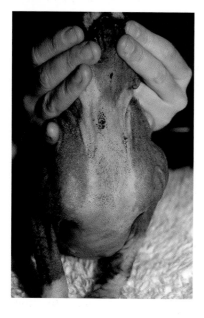

Fig. 1.6 Comedones on neck of Devon Rex cross.

- Skin temperature – may be warm in hyperthyroidism.
- Colour – pallor, erythema, hyperpigmentation.
- Primary and secondary lesions – pustules, papules, comedones (Fig. 1.6).
- Areas of alopecia – has the hair fallen out or has it been nibbled short?

Hair

- Will the hair epilate easily? Is the examination table covered in hair after you have examined the cat?
- Do the hairs look unusual – are there follicular casts?

After taking a careful history and completing a physical and dermatological examination, the clinician should be in a position to compile a list of differential diagnoses. This helps in deciding which further diagnostic tests are required. It is often not necessary to perform every test on each animal. This can also act as a guide to the owners at an early stage as to the possible causes of the disease, the prognosis and what diagnostic investigations are to be undertaken. It is important at this stage to discuss a treatment plan with the owner, including the potential costs.

Diagnostic tests

Initial diagnostic tests

- Wet paper test – the coat is brushed onto a piece of wet paper to identify flea faeces, which show up as red streaks. This should be undertaken in all cases. This is often negative in a cat due to overgrooming, and a negative wet paper test does not preclude fleas.
- Coat brushings onto dry paper can be examined with a hand lens to look for surface parasites, e.g. *Cheyletiella*, lice. Often negative due to the cat's grooming activity. Where possible samples should be taken from inaccessible areas of the cat's body such as the back of the neck.
- Acetate tape impression smears of coat – tape is pressed repeatedly onto the coat to pick up eggs from the hairs as well as parasites on the surface of the skin, e.g. lice, *Trombicula*. Also a useful way to pick up flea faeces.
- Acetate tape impression smears from skin – tape is pressed firmly onto an alopecic area of skin (clipped if necessary). Special stains (Diff Quik) applied to the tape can be used to identify surface bacteria, yeast (especially *Malassezia*).
- Skin scrapings.
  - Deep skin scraping – taken using a scalpel blade to a depth to produce capillary ooze. Material mounted in either 10% potassium hydroxide or liquid paraffin. It is especially important to choose the site appropriately. Always try and avoid areas that have been traumatised by the cat. The skin may be squeezed when taking scrapings for *Demodex* to try and exude mites from the skin. Always take multiple samples. It is often necessary to sedate the cat to perform scrapings.
  - Superficial skin scraping (Fig. 1.7) – *Cheyletiella*, dermatophytes. Scalpel blade is moistened with either 10% potassium hydroxide or liquid paraffin and scraped through the coat and superficial layers of the skin.
- Hair plucking/trichography.
  - This is probably the single most important diagnostic test in assessment of the alopecic cat. It will definitely establish if the hair loss is traumatic due to overgrooming or whether the hairs are falling out due to infectious or metabolic causes (Fig. 1.8). Hair can be mounted in potassium hydroxide, liquid paraffin or lactophenol cotton blue (visualisation of fungal spores).
  - Assessment of hair tip for damage suggestive of self- inflicted trauma (Figs 1.9, 1.10).
  - Assessment of the hair shaft for:

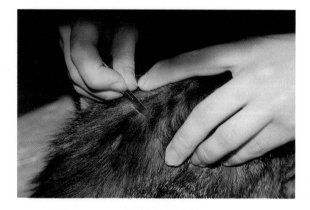

Fig. 1.7 Superficial skin scraping.

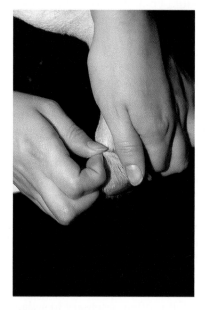

Fig. 1.8 Hair plucking for trichography.

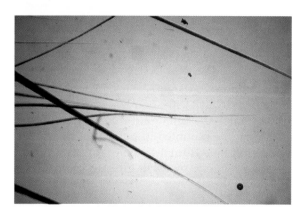

Fig. 1.9 Non-traumatised hair tip in a non-pruritic cat.

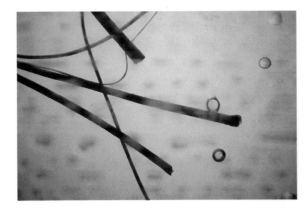

Fig. 1.10 Traumatised hair suggesting excessive grooming.

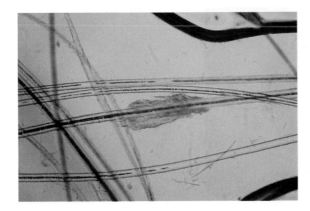

Fig. 1.11 Follicular casts on hair shafts.

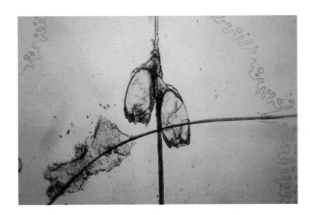

Fig. 1.12 Lice eggs cemented to hair shafts.

Follicular casts – (Fig. 1.11) sebaceous adenitis, steroid administration.
Organisms – (Fig. 1.12) lice eggs, *Demodex*, fungal spores.
Structural abnormalities – (Fig. 1.13) trichorrhexis nodosa.
○ Bulbs – assessment of hair bulbs can be useful.

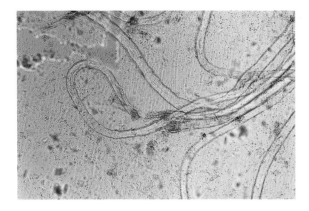

Fig. 1.13 Trichorrhexis nodosa showing 'paint brush-like' splitting of hair shafts.

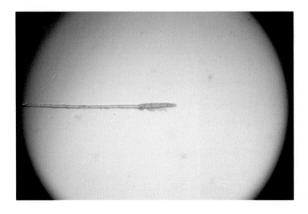

Fig. 1.14 Telogen hair bulbs.

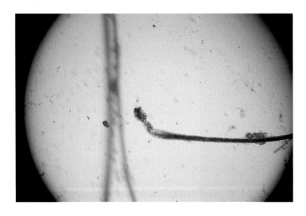

Fig. 1.15 Anogen hair bulbs.

Normal plucking 80–90% hairs are in telogen (Fig. 1.14) and 10–20% of hairs are in anogen (Fig. 1.15).

In metabolic disease where non-traumatic hair loss occurs there is generally an increase in telogen numbers.

○ Fluorescent hairs can be plucked for dermatophyte culture.

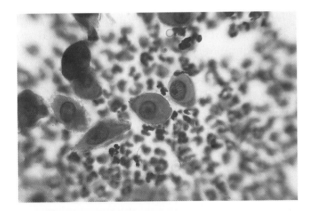

Fig. 1.16 Acanthocytes from a sterile pustule in a case of pemphigus foliaceus.

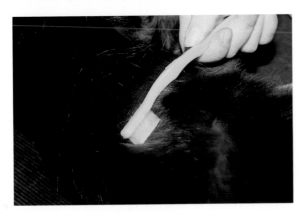

Fig. 1.17 Tooth brushing from coat for dermatophyte culture.

- Impression smears from lesions, e.g. papules, plaques (eosinophilic infiltrate in an eosinophilic granuloma).
- Examination of pustular contents, e.g. bacteria plus degenerate neutrophils seen in bacterial infection; acanthocytes (rounded nucleated keratinocytes), non-degenerate white blood cells (usually neutrophils and eosinophils) in immunological diseases such as pemphigus (Fig. 1.16).
- Fine needle aspirates, especially nodules in neoplastic and pyogranulomatous disease, taken by the following technique:
  - ○ Aspirate taken using 20–21 gauge needle and 5–10 ml syringe.
  - ○ The needle is introduced into the lesion and gentle suction is applied by withdrawing the syringe plunger.
  - ○ The needle can be redirected into different areas of the mass before reapplying suction.
  - ○ Suction is released and the needle is withdrawn from the lesion.
  - ○ Needle and syringe are separated, air is drawn into the syringe, needle is reattached, and contents of syringe and needle are expelled onto a glass slide.
- Sterile toothbrush, hairbrush or carpet square coat brushing for fungal culture (Fig. 1.17).

- ○ Due to the wide range of clinical presentations of dermatophytosis ringworm examination/cultures should be undertaken in any longhaired cat (especially Persians) and in all inflammatory skin diseases.
- ○ The brush is pulled throughout the hair coat collecting scale and hair. It is then submitted to an experienced technician for culture in-house using dermatophyte test medium (DTM) or is submitted to a laboratory.
- ○ It is impossible to assess which dermatophyte has been grown on DTM as reverse pigment and macroconidia are not formed.
- ○ The sample should not be stored in plastic (a paper envelope is best) as this will encourage commensal overgrowth.
- Examination of ear wax.
  - ○ Plain wax rolled onto a microscope slide to look for *Otodectes, Demodex*.
  - ○ Wax stained with Diff Quik to look for cell types and micro-organisms.

Further diagnostic tests

Initial investigations will give information as to which further tests are deemed necessary. It is important to discuss these again with the owner at this stage.

Dermatological tests

- Culture from swabs.
  - ○ Bacterial culture.
    Bacterial infection in the cat tends to be deep/pyogranulomatous. The initial source of the infection will usually give a clue as to whether culture is necessary.
    When the primary insult is a bite forming an abscess, empirical antibiotic therapy can be prescribed based on the bacterial flora of the cat's mouth (see Chapter 2).
    In pyogranulomatous disease aerobic/anaerobic culture should be undertaken to include sensitivity. It is important to inform the laboratory if you are suspicious of an unusual or zoonotic organism, e.g. *Nocardia* or mycobacteria. The help of specialised laboratories may be sought for more unusual or dangerous pathogens.
  - ○ Fungal culture.
    Dermatophyte culture has already been described (see above), although tissue culture (see below) is usually the culture method of choice for deep fungal infections.
    Samples of exudate taken from deep within the draining tract can be diagnostic in diseases such as sporotrichosis.
  - ○ Yeast, especially *Malassezia* – contact plates/swab.
- Tissue culture taken as a biopsy sample, for deeper lesions for both fungal and bacterial culture. Submitted to the laboratory in appropriate transport medium.
- Biopsy – punch biopsy ideally of primary lesions or excisional biopsy of, e.g. nodules.
  - ○ Indications for biopsy include:
    Suspected neoplastic lesions.

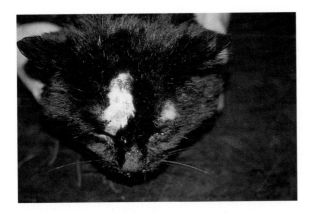

Fig. 1.18 Ulcerative lesion on head of cat with a fibrosarcoma.

Ulcerative/vesicular lesions (Fig. 1.18). Where an ulcer is biopsied aim to include a margin of normal skin.

Skin disease unresponsive to rational therapy.

Unusual or serious skin disease, especially when the cat is systemically unwell.

To make a diagnosis in a disease where expensive or potentially dangerous drugs are to be used.

○ A biopsy should not be performed as a means of avoiding a proper work–up or as a short cut to a diagnosis.

○ Multiple biopsies should always be taken, where possible from a variety of different lesions, at different stages of development.

- Allergy testing – *in vivo* tests.
  ○ These are difficult to perform and read in the cat, and should only be undertaken by an experienced clinician.
- Trial therapy.
  ○ Antiparasitic therapy – in cases of suspected flea allergic dermatitis.
  ○ Antibiotics – in pustular disease to assess if infectious or sterile disease.
  ○ Food trial – where a diet is suspected as a cause of the disease – food allergy.
  ○ Drug withdrawal – drug eruptions.
  ○ Trial therapy with anti-inflammatory therapy is rarely, if ever, warranted in the cat.

General

- A routine screen should include – haematology, biochemistry, thyroid levels, feline leukaemia virus (FeLV), feline immunodeficiency virus (FIV).
- Dynamic function tests – ACTH stimulation test, low/high dose dexamethasone suppression test, TSH/TRH stimulation test. See Chapter 8 for suggested protocols.
- Ultrasonography – visualisation of adrenal glands, pancreatic architecture in pancreatic neoplastic syndrome.

- X-rays – especially of chest in cases of metastatic bronchial carcinoma, thymoma.
- Electrocardiogram (ECG) – cardiac abnormalities seen with hyperthyroidism.

Once a diagnosis has been made it is important to again discuss with the owner the long-term prognosis for the animal, the success rate for the therapy, the cost and the length of course of the treatment. Owners are also more comfortable if their pet's condition has a name, so write it down for them.

Often in feline cases the best form of therapy for the cat cannot be undertaken. Many cats are impossible to give tablets, shampoo, or inject on a regular basis. Such factors will inevitably influence your therapy. If a short course of drugs is required for a long-term resolution of the problem, many owners are prepared to struggle. If the cat needs to be on therapy for the rest of its life, then owners may be quite reasonably less compliant. It is possible that a surgical option will be more attractive than medical therapy. It is also important to discuss with the owner the long-term prognosis for the cat if the disease isn't treated. Alopecia without inflammation caused by atopy may look unsightly but may be a tolerable option rather than monthly desensitising vaccines. This procedure can often take as long as the initial consultation but is as important. If the owner appreciates what you have done and why you have done it, then long-term client compliance is much better.

Chapter 2

Bacterial Skin Diseases

General

Bacterial skin infection in the cat is rare. Subcutaneous abscesses are the most common forms of infection, usually due to bite wounds. Feline superficial and deep infections are almost always associated with other underlying disease processes such as metabolic or immunological abnormalities.

The primary pathogen in superficial infections is *Staphylococcus intermedius*. In deep pyoderma many different aerobic and anaerobic bacteria including *Pasteurella multocida*, β-haemolytic streptococcus, *Actinomyces* spp. *Bacteroides* spp. and *Fusobacterium* spp. can be identified.

Pyoderma can be classified according to depth:

- Surface.
- Superficial.
- Deep.

SURFACE PYODERMA

Definition

Infection involving the outermost layers of the epidermis.

Types

- Acute moist dermatitis.
- Intertrigo complex.

Acute moist dermatitis

Underlying causes

- Site of traumatisation can give a clue to the underlying cause.
  - Allergy – atopy (Fig. 2.1), food, fleas.
  - Ectoparasites.
  - Internal disease urolithiasis, abdominal foreign body (e.g. fur balls) (Fig. 2.2).

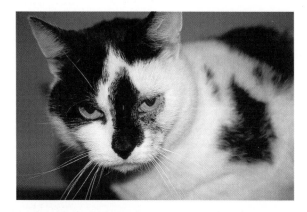

Fig. 2.1 Acute moist dermatitis caused through face rubbing in an allergic cat.

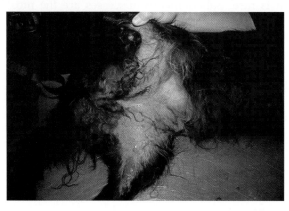

Fig. 2.2 Acute moist dermatitis caused by licking due to urolithiasis.

- ○ Hyperthermia secondary to hyperthyroidism.
- ○ Trauma – bites, injection reactions.
- ○ Psychogenic – flanks or tail (especially in oriental breeds).

Clinical signs

- Localised area of moist erythematous exudation.
- Margins are clearly defined; lesion is surrounded by halo of erythematous skin.

Differential diagnosis

- Eosinophilic granuloma.
- Deep localised pyoderma.
- Dermatophytosis.
- Neoplasia (especially squamous cell carcinoma).
- Ulcerative dermatitis with linear subepidermal fibrosis.

Diagnosis

- History especially important with internal disease.
- Skin scrapes.

- Impression smear – Diff Quik stains reveal neutrophils, eosinophils and bacteria.
- Fungal culture

Treatment

- Check and correct any underlying causes where possible.
- Clip area (sedation usually necessary).
- Collar or bandage to allow healing and break itch–scratch cycle.

Topical therapy

- Antibacterial shampoos – especially those containing chlorhexidine (Duoderma, C.Vet, Malaseb, Leo Labs). Benzoyl peroxide and iodine products can be irritating to cats.
- Topical antibiotics – 2% mupirocin cream.
- Topical antibiotic and steroid combinations (for short-term use only) – fusidic acid/betamethasone gel (Fuciderm, Leo Labs).

Systemic therapy

- Should not be used when internal disease is suspected.
- Short acting steroids, e.g. prednisolone 1–2 mg/kg once or twice daily for 7–10 days.

INTERTRIGO COMPLEX (SKIN FOLD PYODERMA)

- Dermatitis caused by friction between two closely apposed areas of skin.
- Multiplication of commensal organisms leads to disease.
- Bacteria and yeasts can be identified.

Types

- Facial fold.
- Body fold.
- Interdigital/nail fold.

Facial fold pyoderma

- Breed incidence – Persians (Fig. 2.3), other short faced breeds.
- Check for primary eye disease, e.g. infectious or allergic conjunctivitis leading to ocular discharge.

Clinical signs

- Exudation and crusting with erythema, in the early stages confined to the intertriginous areas.

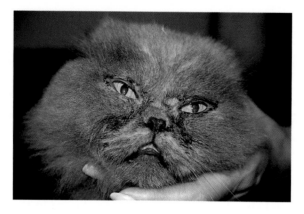

Fig. 2.3 Facial fold pyoderma in a Persian cat.

Diagnosis

- Clinical appearance.
- Acetate tape impression smear stained with Diff Quik to identify yeasts (*Malassezia*) or bacteria (*Staphylococcus*).
- Skin scrapings.

Treatment

- Correction of any primary eye disease.
- Surgical therapy not usually an option.
- Topical therapy as acute moist dermatitis.

Body fold pyoderma

- Obese cats, animals with mammary hyperplasia due to hormonal therapy or lactation.

Clinical signs/diagnosis

- As facial fold.

Treatment

- Medical therapy as acute moist dermatitis.
- Weight reduction, correction of mammary hyperplasia.

Interdigital/nail fold pyoderma

- Can occur due to overgrooming in allergic or seborrhoeic cats.
- *Malassezia* (Fig. 2.4) and bacteria can be involved.

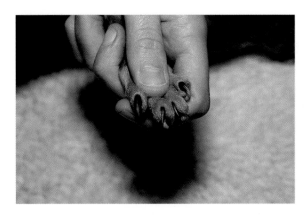

Fig. 2.4 Nail fold *Malassezia* in a Devon Rex.

Clinical signs

- Erythema, often with a malodorous seborrhoeic discharge.

Diagnosis

- As facial fold.

Treatment

- Bacterial component – as for acute moist dermatitis.
- Where *Malassezia* identified:
  - Gentle anti-seborrhoeic shampoo containing sulphur, selenium sulphide (Seleen, Sanofi).
  - Topical anti-yeast products containing miconazole, e.g. Malaseb shampoo (Leo Labs).

SUPERFICIAL BACTERIAL INFECTION

Definition

- Bacterial infection that involves the epidermis and intact follicle.
- Rare condition in the cat.

Types

- Impetigo.
- Folliculitis.
- Dermatophilosis.

Impetigo

- Subcorneal pustules most obvious in sparsely haired areas.

Cause and pathogenesis

- Juvenile impetigo – bacteria involved include *Staphylococcus*, *Pasteurella multocida* or β-haemolytic streptococcus.
  - ○ Overgrooming of kittens by queen.
- Adult onset impetigo – bacteria as juvenile form.
  - ○ Viral immunosuppression, e.g. FeLV, FIV, pox virus.
  - ○ Debilitating disease, e.g. neoplasia.
  - ○ Endocrine disease, e.g. hyperadrenocorticism.
  - ○ Allergy, especially atopy (Fig. 2.5).

Clinical signs

- Non-follicular pustules, rupture to form papules and crusts; pruritus variable.
- Distribution can be generalised but often seen on hairless ventral abdominal areas (Fig. 2.6).

Differential diagnosis

- Miliary dermatitis
- Dermatophytosis

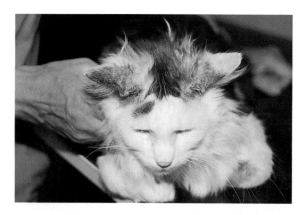

Fig. 2.5 Adult onset impetigo on the ear secondary to atopy.

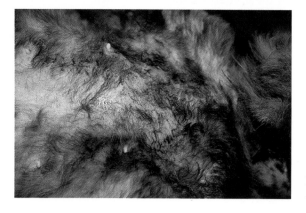

Fig. 2.6 Impetigo on ventral abdomen.

Diagnosis

- History – especially important in adult onset disease.
- Clinical signs.
- Skin scrapings.
- Fungal culture – as a rule out.
- Cytology of lesions.
  - Degenerate neutrophils with bacteria.
  - Eosinophils usually uncommon.
- Culture and sensitivity.
- Identification of underlying diseases where appropriate.

Treatment

- Identification and treatment of underlying cause where necessary.
- Antibiotics based on culture and sensitivity.
- Treatment may be life-long where immunosuppression cannot be treated, e.g. FIV.

Bacterial folliculitis

- Bacterial infection of the intact hair follicle causes formation of follicular pustules.

Cause and pathogenesis

- Bacteria involved include *Staphylococcus* (both coagulase positive and negative), *Pasteurella multocida* or β-haemolytic streptococcus.
- Underlying causes – as adult onset impetigo.

Clinical signs

- Follicular pustules and papules progressing to crusting and alopecia usually located on the face, neck (Fig. 2.7) and head.
- Appearance of non-allergic miliary dermatitis

Differential diagnosis

- Allergic miliary dermatitis.
- Dermatophytosis.
- Demodicosis.

Diagnosis and treatment

- As impetigo

Dermatophilosis

- Rare superficial crusting dermatosis caused by *Dermatophilus congolensis.*

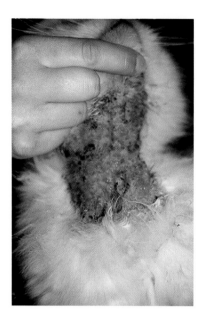

Fig. 2.7 Bacterial folliculitis on ventral neck secondary to atopy.

Cause and pathogenesis

- Infection thought to come from carrier animals, especially farm animals and horses.

Predisposing factors

- Moisture required for zoospore release.
- Skin damage necessary to allow spore penetration, e.g. ectoparasites, fight wound.

Clinical signs

- Can affect both haired and glabrous skin, also deeper infections of skin and lymph nodes.
- Superficial skin lesions – painful commonly on dorsum shoulder and thigh; also face, ears and feet.
- Early lesions – papules and pustules later form crusts.
- Typical 'paint brush' lesions – exudative purulent dermatitis with crusts containing embedded hairs.

Differential diagnosis

- Dermatophytosis.
- Allergic miliary dermatitis.
- Pox virus.
- Other bacterial infections.

Diagnosis

- History of contact with carrier animals.
- Clinical signs.
- Direct smear of underside of crust stained with Diff Quik – parallel rows of Gram-positive cocci look like 'railroad tracks'.
- Culture and sensitivity (crusts and exudate).
- Skin scrapings.
- Fungal culture – as a rule out.
- Skin biopsy useful in chronic cases.

Treatment

- Identification of carrier animals and removal of predisposing factors.
- Systemic antibiotics based on culture and sensitivity. Ampicillin, cephalosporins and lincomycin can be used for empirical therapy (see Table 2.1).
- Sedation and removal of crusts with mild anti-seborrhoeic shampoo may be useful.

DEEP BACTERIAL INFECTIONS

- Infection of the deeper tissues of the dermis and often sub cutis.
- Do not occur spontaneously.
- An underlying predisposing cause should always be sought.

Localised deep pyoderma

- Infection is confined to a small area.
- This is the most common form of pyoderma in the cat, forming a subcutaneous abscess.

Predisposing factors

These include:

- Bites.
- Wounds.
- Foreign bodies.

Cause and pathogenesis

- Usually caused by bite wounds (Fig. 2.8). Small puncture wound injects bacteria into the skin.
- Bacteria involved are usually those of feline oral cavity, i.e. *Pasteurella multocida*, β-haemolytic streptococcus, *Bacteroides* and fusiform bacilli.
- The wound heals rapidly and a local infection develops over 48–72 hours.

Table 2.1 Systemic antibacterial therapy

Antibiotic	Dose rate	Indications
Amikacin*	5–10 mg/kg s.c. every 12 hours	Gram-negative rods, atypical mycobacteria, *M. avium*
Amoxycillin	11–22 mg/kg p.o. every 8–12 hours	Cat bite abscesses
Ampicillin	20 mg/kg p.o. every 6–12 hours	*Actinomyces, Nocardia, Dermatophilus*
Cephalexin	25 mg/kg p.o. every 12 hours	*Nocardia, Dermatophilus*
Clavamox (amoxycillin/ clavulanate)	12.5–25 mg/kg p.o. every 8–12 hours	Cat bite abscesses, staphylococcal infections
Clindamycin	5.5 mg/kg p.o. every 12 hours	*Nocardia*, cat bite abscesses, staphylococcal infections
Clofazimine	2–12 mg/kg p.o. every 12 hours; long courses up to 6 months required	Feline leprosy
Enroflaxacin	5.0 mg/kg p.o. every 12 hours	Gram-negative rods, atypical mycobacteria, *M. avium*, staphylococcal infections
Lincomycin	22 mg/kg p.o. every 12 hours	Staphylococcal infections, *Dermatophilus*
Penicillin G procaine	10–15 mg/kg i.m. or s.c. every 12 hours	Actinomyces
Potentiated sulphonamides (trimethoprim/ sulphonamide)	Dose is mg of total product: 30 mg/kg p.o. every 12 hours	*Actinobacillus, Nocardia*
Rifampin†	5 mg/kg p.o. every 24 hours	Feline leprosy
Streptomycin	10 mg/kg i.m. or s.c. every 24 hours	*Actinobacillus*, plague
Tetracycline	10–22 mg/kg p.o. every 8–12 hours	*Actinomyces*, L-form bacteria, plague

Key: p.o., by mouth; i.m., intramuscularly; s.c., subcutaneously.
*Nephrotoxic drug – monitor renal function.
†Heptotoxic drug – monitor hepatic function.

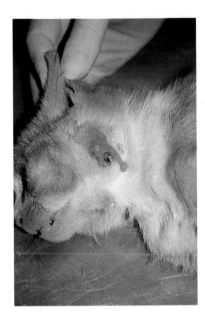

Fig. 2.8 Bite wound on the side of the face.

Clinical signs

- Swollen area covered only by a small crust.
- Common sites – tail base, shoulder and neck.
- Area warm and painful.

Differential diagnosis

- Other less common bacterial infections including:
  - Mycobacteria.
  - *Yersinia pestis.*
  - *Nocardia* spp.
  - *Actinomyces* spp.
- Fungal mycetoma.
- Neoplasia.

Diagnosis

- Clinical appearance.
- Response to therapy.

Treatment

- Surgical drainage (sedation is often required).
- Flushing of the abscess with saline or chlorhexidine solution.
- Antibiotics 5–10 days. Amoxycillin, clindamycin can be used for empirical therapy (see Table 2.1).

- Uncomplicated localised abscesses should heal uneventfully with appropriate therapy.
- If there is failure to heal an immunosuppressive factor should be sought or other differentials explored.

Generalised deep infections

- Involve larger areas, i.e. an extensive region, e.g. face.
- Predisposing factors include:
  - Systemic disease causing immunosuppression, e.g. viral infection, neoplasia.
  - Inappropriate therapy with hormones (especially progestagens) or glucocorticoids.
- In all cases of generalised pyoderma where several sites are involved the cat has a second disease which must be identified.

Cause and pathogenesis

- Usually caused by trauma to the skin, e.g. fight wounds, road traffic accidents, parasite damage (Fig. 2.9).
- Bacterial flora similar to localised deep infection.

Clinical signs

- Extensive area of swelling with exudation and often fistula formation (Fig. 2.10).
- Area warm and painful.
- Cat systemically unwell.

Differential diagnosis

- As localised deep infection.

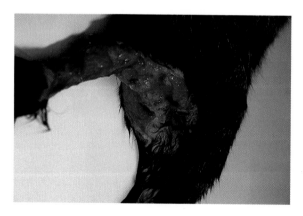

Fig. 2.9 Deep cellulitis secondary to fly strike.

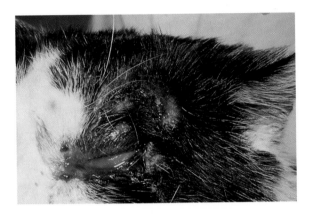

Fig. 2.10 Periocular cellulitis in an immunosuppressed cat (picture courtesy of P. Boydell).

Diagnosis

- Clinical appearance.
- Cytology of lesions stained with Diff Quik.
- Tissue culture – to include both aerobic and anaerobic cultures.
- Routine blood profile to include FeLV and FIV.

Treatment

- Antibiotics for a minimum of 3–4 weeks based on appropriate culture and sensitivity.
- Therapy of any underlying immunosuppressive factors.

UNCOMMON PYOGRANULOMATOUS BACTERIAL INFECTIONS

- Bacterial pseudomycetoma.
- Actinomycosis.
- Actinobacillosis.
- Nocardiosis.
- Plague.
- L-Form infections.
- Mycobacterial infections.
  - Cutaneous tuberculosis.
  - Opportunistic mycobacteria.
  - Feline leprosy.

Bacterial pseudomycetoma

- Chronic pyogranulomatous disease caused by non-branching bacteria.

Cause and pathogenesis

- Usually coagulase positive staphylococci, also *Pseudomonas* sp., *Streptococcus* sp., and *Proteus* sp. Mixed infections can be found.
- Infection introduced by trauma, especially bites, wounds or penetrating foreign body.
- Pyogranuloma forms as host contains, but does not eliminate, infection.

Clinical signs

- Firm cutaneous nodules – single or multiple; bone or muscle can be involved.
- Draining fistulae – exudate contains white tissue grains.
- Any site, especially extremities.

Differential diagnosis

Other bacterial infections including:

- Mycobacteria.
- *Yersinia pestis* (plague).
- Actinomycosis.
- Actinobacillosis.
- Nocardiosis.

As well as:

- Dermatophytic pseudomycetoma.
- Fungal mycetoma.
- Neoplasia.
- Foreign body.

Diagnosis

- Exudative cytology, neutrophils and macrophages with bacteria.
- Skin biopsy – including special bacterial and fungal stains.
- Tissue culture for both bacteria and fungi.

Treatment

- Surgical drainage and antimicrobial therapy based on culture and sensitivity are rarely effective.
- Surgical excision often requiring amputation of the limb is most effective.

Actinomycosis

- Rare pyogranulomatous and/or suppurative disease caused by Gram-positive anaerobic filamentous *Actinomyces* organisms.

Cause and pathogenesis

- Opportunistic commensals of the gastrointestinal tract.
- Infection caused through trauma, e.g. bite wounds.

Clinical signs

- Insidious onset of lesions up to 2 years after initial injury.
- Painful subcutaneous abscesses occur at any site.
- Draining tracts common – sulphur granules seen in 50% of cases.
- Discharge thick yellow–grey – thin haemorrhagic, usually malodorous.
- Osteomyelitis and empyema may occur.

Differential diagnosis

- As bacterial pseudomycetoma, especially nocardiosis.

Diagnosis

- Clinical signs.
- Direct smear of fine needle aspirate – Gram stain.
- Anaerobic culture.
- Biopsy using special stains.

Treatment

- Surgical excision has highest success rate.
- Debulk with prolonged antibiosis in inaccessible sites.
- Useful drugs include penicillin, ampicillin and tetracycline (see Table 2.1).
- Treatment for minimum 1 month beyond remission, usually 3–4 months in total.

Actinbacillosis

- Rare pyogranulomatous disease caused by Gram-negative aerobic coccobacillus *Actinobacillus lignieresii.*

Cause and pathogenesis

- Commensal oral cavity, does not survive in the environment.
- Infection follows traumatic lesions, especially bites.

Clinical signs

- Lesions insidious onset, weeks–months.
- Painful single or multiple thick-walled abscesses.
- Lesions found on head, neck, mouth and limbs.
- Odourless thick white–green discharge with yellow sulphur granules.

Differential diagnosis

- As bacterial pseudomycetoma.

Diagnosis

- Clinical signs.
- Direct smears of purulent discharge.
- Aerobic cultures.
- Biopsy with special stains.

Treatment

- Surgical excision where possible.
- Medical therapy – drain and flush area plus antibiotics.
- Antibiotics based on culture and sensitivity.
- Useful drugs include sodium iodide (20 mg/kg orally twice daily) or potentiated sulphonamides (see Table 2.1).
- Treatment for 1 month beyond remission.
- Relapses common, guarded prognosis.

Nocardiosis

- Rare pyogranulomatous and/or suppurative infection caused by Gram-positive, partially acid fast branching filamentous aerobe *Nocardia* sp., especially *N. asteroides*.

Cause and pathogenesis

- Soil saprophytes.
- Infection by wound contamination, especially bites plus ingestion and inhalation.
- Common in immunosuppressed animals.

Clinical signs

- Cutaneous lesions similar to actinomycosis.
- Painful subcutaneous abscesses, nodules and cellulitis.
- Discharge thick yellow–grey – thin haemorrhagic usually malodorous.
- Lesions common on limbs and feet (Fig. 2.11), also ventral abdomen.
- Systemic signs – pyothorax, weakness, anorexia, pyrexia, and neurological signs.

Differential diagnosis

- As bacterial pseudomycetoma, especially actinomycosis.

Diagnosis

- Clinical signs.
- Direct smear of fine needle aspirate – Gram stain.
- Aerobic culture.

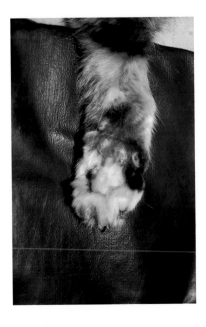

Fig. 2.11 *Nocardia* infection on the footpad.

- Biopsy with special stains.
- Investigation of potential underlying immunosuppression should include blood samples for FeLV, FIV.
- Where systemic signs are present investigation should include appropriate X-rays, ultrasound, etc.

Treatment

- Surgical drainage.
- Antibiotics based on culture and sensitivity.
- Useful drugs include potentiated sulphonamides, ampicillin combined with cephalosporin or clindamycin.
- Treatment for 1 month after remission, up to 3–4 months in total.
- Prognosis guarded, especially if cat immunosuppressed.

Plague

- Rare disease caused by facultative anaerobic Gram-negative coccobacillus *Yersinia pestis.*
- Public health risk.

Cause and pathogenesis

- Non-motile non-spore forming organism.
- Three forms recognised – bubonic, pneumonic and septicaemic plague.

- Incubation period
  - 1–2 days by ingestion or inhalation
  - 2–6 days by flea bite, penetrating wound or mucous membrane.
- Cats usually infected by rodent fleas.
- Humans become infected by cats bringing home fleas or dead rodents, or from feline body fluids, e.g. pus, saliva.

Clinical signs

- 50% of cases are bubonic plague.
- Localised abscesses occur near infection site, especially head and neck.
- Pyrexia, anorexia, depression – up to 75% mortality.

Differential diagnosis

- As bacterial pseudomycetoma +.
- Wound infections.
- Cat abscesses.

Diagnosis

- Clinical signs.
- Culture of exudate.
- Immunofluorescence of impression smears.

Treatment

- Prompt therapy important due to rapid and fatal progression of the disease.
- Local abscesses lanced, drained and flushed with care.
- Antibiotics based on culture and sensitivity where possible.
- Useful drugs include tetracycline and streptomycin.

L-Form infections

Cause and pathogenesis

- Rare disease caused by bacteria that are partially cell-wall deficient similar to *Mycoplasma*.
- Cannot be cultured routinely.

Clinical signs

- Systemic signs – pyrexia, depressed, polyarthropathy.
- Cutaneous signs – abscesses, exudate non-odorous, often over joints.

Differential diagnosis

- As bacterial pseudomycetoma.

Diagnosis

- Clinical signs.
- Culture unsuccessful.
- Electron microscopy of fresh tissue reveals organisms.

Treatment

- Complete response seen to tetracycline.

MYCOBACTERIAL INFECTIONS

- Cutaneous tuberculosis
  - *Mycobacterium bovis*
  - *M. tuberculosis*
  - *M. avium*
- Opportunistic mycobacteria
  - *M. chelonei*
  - *M. fortuitum*
  - and others
- Feline leprosy
  - *M. lepraemurium*

Cutaneous tuberculosis

- Rare mycobacterial infection.

Cause and pathogenesis

- *M. bovis* and *M. tuberculosis* passed from processed meat or milk, or from infected humans.
- *M. avium* environmental saprophyte. Siamese may be predisposed.

Clinical signs

- Systemic signs – respiratory and gastrointestinal signs most common.
- Anorexia, lymphadenopathy and pyrexia.
- Cutaneous lesions – variable; ulcers, abscesses, plaques and nodules can all occur.
- Discharge malodorous yellow/green – no tissue grains.
- Lesions found on head, neck and limbs.

Differential diagnosis

- Other infectious pyogranulomas, e.g. nocardiosis, actinomycosis, atypical mycobacteria, feline leprosy.

- Eumycotic mycetoma.
- Dermatophytic mycetoma.
- Neoplasia.
- Foreign body granuloma.

Diagnosis

- History.
- Radiography of chest.
- Biopsy, including special stain for mycobacteria (Ziehl Neelson).
- Culture – special media required.
- Lymphocyte blastogenesis test.

Treatment

- *M. bovis* and *M. tuberculosis* – euthanasia recommended due to public health risk.
- *M. avium*
  - Antibiotic therapy on the basis of culture and sensitivity. Empirical therapy may be useful with amikacin (see Table 2.1).
  - Surgical removal or cryosurgery of lesions is less successful – recurrence common.

Opportunistic mycobacterial infections

- Uncommon granulomatous disease caused by atypical mycobacteria.

Cause and pathogenesis

- Free-living organisms, usually found in soil, and artificial and natural water sources.
- Usually harmless but can be facultative pathogens.
- *M. fortuitum* and *M. chelonei* most commonly isolated from feline cases.
- Infection introduced through traumatic events such as bites.

Clinical signs

- Cutaneous lesions develop over several weeks: can present as non-healing wounds.
- Abscesses form with ulceration and draining fistulae (Fig. 2.12).
- Most commonly found caudal abdomen, lower back and pelvic areas.
- Pain and lymphadenopathy variable.
- Systemic signs rare.

Differential diagnosis

- As cutaneous tuberculosis.

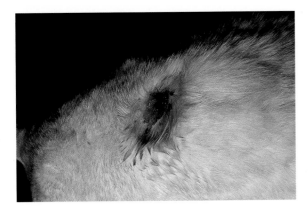

Fig. 2.12 Atypical mycobacteria infection on flank.

Diagnosis

- History.
- Clinical signs.
- Fine needle aspirate of closed lesions.
- Cultures grow rapidly on a variety of different media.
- Biopsy including special stains, e.g. Ziehl Neelson.

Treatment

- Spontaneous resolution rare.
- Any treatment carries a guarded prognosis.
- Wide surgical excision with debridement and systemic antibiotics based on culture and sensitivity where possible. Empirical therapy may be useful with enrofloxacin or amikacin (see Table 2.1).

Feline leprosy

- Granulomatous infection caused by acid fast organism.

Cause and pathogenesis

- Infection caused by a poorly characterised mycobacterium.
- Agent is difficult to culture and only identified on stained biopsy sections.
- Thought to be caused by *M. lepraemurium.*

Clinical signs

- Usually young cats.
- Non-painful lesions – single or multiple nodules, often non-healing fistulae.
- Usually found on head or extremities.
- Lesions enlarge but do not spread.
- Cat systemically well.

Differential diagnosis

- As cutaneous tuberculosis.

Diagnosis

- History.
- Clinical signs.
- Presence of acid fast bacilli on direct smears and biopsy material.
- Cutaneous tuberculosis should be ruled out by guinea pig inoculation.

Treatment

- Surgical removal successful for single or well circumscribed lesions.
- Cryosurgery useful in some cases.
- Medical treatment variable success based on empirical therapy. Useful drugs include clofazimine or rifampin (see Table 2.1).

Chapter 3

Investigation and Management of Dermatophytosis

Dermatophytosis

Cause and pathogenesis

- Usually caused by *Microsporum canis*, *Microsporum gypseum*, *Trichophyton mentagrophytes*.
- *M. canis* is the most common cause of dermatophytosis in cats.
- Zoonotic infection.
- Transmission occurs from:
  - Infected animal (hair, scale).
  - Environmental contamination (housing, heating vents).
  - Fomites (grooming equipment, bedding).
- Sources of infection:
  - *M. canis* – zoophilic dermatophyte. Reservoir – usually cats.
  - *T. mentagrophytes* – zoophilic dermatophyte. Reservoir – rodents.
  - *M. gypseum* – geophilic dermatophyte. Reservoir – soil.
  - *T. erinacei* – zoophilic dermatophyte. Reservoir – hedgehogs.
  - *M. persicolor* – zoophilic dermatophyte. Reservoir – small rodents.

Predisposing factors

- Cell mediated immunity is important for defence mechanism.
- Factors affecting this predispose to infection.
  - Young animals – delayed development of immunity and local skin mechanisms.
  - Viral infection, e.g. FIV, FeLV.
  - Neoplasia.
  - Poor nutrition.
  - Anti-inflammatory/immunosuppressive drug therapy, especially progestagens.
  - Pregnancy/lactation.
  - Systemic disease, e.g. hyperadrenocorticism, diabetes mellitus.
- Ectoparasitic disease (especially fleas and *Cheyletiella*) causes trauma to the skin to allow fungal spores to establish.

Clinical signs

- Can mimic many different feline dermatoses – dependent on the type of dermatophyte and host immune status.
- Typical lesions – areas of alopecia with fine grey scale (Fig. 3.1), found on head, pinnae and paws.
- Can also appear as:
  - ○ Comedone formation.
  - ○ Non-allergic miliary dermatitis – widespread papulocrustous dermatitis (Fig. 3.2).
  - ○ Diffuse alopecia often with crusting (Fig. 3.3).
  - ○ Exfoliative erythroderma (Fig. 3.4).
  - ○ Generalised seborrhoea (Fig. 3.5).
  - ○ Chin folliculitis.
  - ○ Fungal kerion – erythematous exudative area of furunculosis.
  - ○ Pseudomycetoma seen in Persian cats appears as ulcerated, discharging subcutaneous nodules, especially on trunk and at tail base (Fig. 3.6).
  - ○ Onychomycosis – rare.

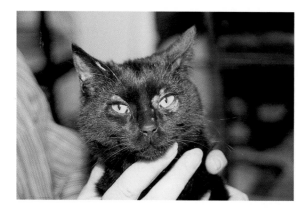

Fig. 3.1 Typical periocular grey crusting seen with *M. canis* infection.

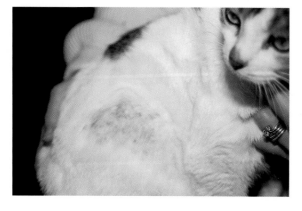

Fig. 3.2 Widespread papulocrustous dermatitis due to *M. canis*.

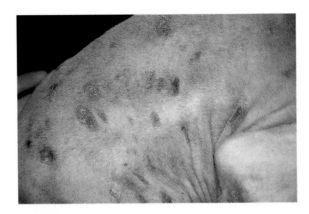

Fig. 3.3 Diffuse alopecia with macular areas of hyperpigmentation caused by *M. canis*.

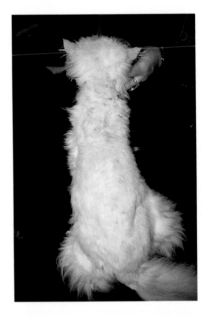

Fig. 3.4 Exfoliative erythroderma due to *M. canis*.

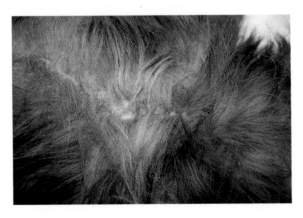

Fig. 3.5 Generalised seborrhoea due to *M. canis*.

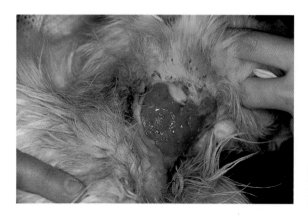

Fig. 3.6 Pseudomycetoma in a Persian cat (picture courtesy R. Bond).

Differential diagnosis

- Dermatophytosis can mimic any feline skin disease so should be considered in every dermatological case.

Diagnosis

General assessment of skin to check for concurrent disease

- Wet paper test for fleas.
- Superficial and deep skin scrapings for ectoparasites.

Dermatophytosis

- Woods's lamp – apple green fluorescence on individually plucked hair shafts.
  - ○ Only 50% of *M. canis* infections fluoresce.
  - ○ False negatives – Woods's lamp not warmed up; fluorescence destroyed by topical medications.
  - ○ False positives – bacterial infection (not apple green fluorescence); topical medication.
- Microscopy of plucked hairs in 10% potassium hydroxide or mineral oil shows presence of arthrospores.
- Fungal culture.
  - ○ Animal – MacKenzie method. Sterile toothbrush brushed through coat then implanted into culture medium. Dermatophyte test medium (DTM) or Sabourauds dextrose agar (Figs 3.7–3.10).
  - ○ Environment – sample as above from soft furnishings, carpets, cages, window ledges, etc.
  - ○ False negatives on DTM – some isolates produce no colour change.
  - ○ False positives on DTM – saprophytic fungi cause colour changes.
  - ○ Identification of the type of dermatophyte is useful in order to establish the initial source of the problem. A dermatophyte may be grown on DTM to

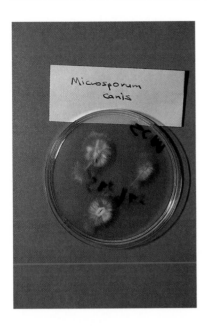

Fig. 3.7 Colony morphology *M. canis* on Sabouraud's dextrose agar.

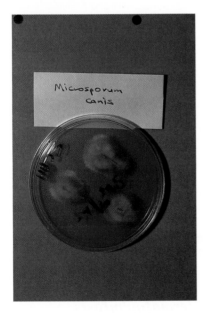

Fig. 3.8 Reverse pigment *M. canis* on Sabouraud's dextrose agar.

establish its presence and then subcultured onto Sabouraud's dextrose agar to identify the macroconidia, microconidia, colony morphology and reverse pigment (Figs 3.11–3.14, Table 3.1).
- Biopsy with special stains.

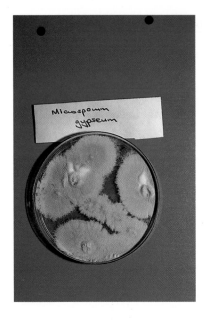

Fig. 3.9 Colony morphology *M. gypseum* on Sabouraud's dextrose agar.

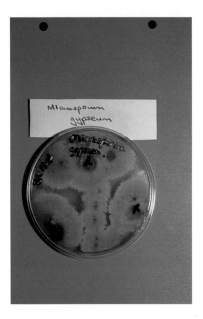

Fig. 3.10 Reverse pigment *M. gypseum* on Sabouraud's dextrose agar.

Treatment of individual animals with dermatophytosis

- Dermatophytosis will often resolve without treatment. However, because of the risk of owner contagion and reinfection via fomites and other animals, treatment is indicated.
- Routine ectoparasite control should be performed in all cases, e.g. fipronil (Merial).

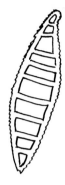

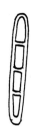

Fig. 3.12 Line diagram macroconidia *T. mentagrophytes.*

Fig. 3.11 Line diagram macroconidia *M. canis.*

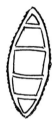

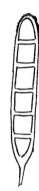

Fig. 3.13 Line diagram macroconidia *M. gypseum.*

Fig. 3.14 Line diagram macroconidia *M. persicolor.*

Animal

Topical treatment

- Localised lesions.
  - ○ Gentle clipping (cat may need to be sedated) with no. 10 blade, not a surgical clip.
  - ○ Lotion or cream containing miconazole, clotrimazole applied twice daily up to 6 cm beyond active edge of the lesion.
  - ○ At present no topical products are licensed for use in cats.
- Generalised lesions.
  - ○ Whole body clip (probably not necessary if animal can be shampooed adequately).
  - ○ Shampoo whole body twice weekly – suitable products contain chlorhexidine, miconazole, (Malaseb, Leo Labs), enilconazole, (Imaverol, Janssen).

Table 3.1 Dermatophytes colony and microscopic morphology

Species	Culture characteristics on Sabouraud's dextrose agar			Appearance of macroconidia	Microconidia
	From	Colour	Reverse pigment		
M. canis	Initial growth cotton wool-like then powdery with central depression	White–buff	Yellow/orange later, orange/brown	Abundant, spindle shaped, curved tip. Thick spinous walls contain 6–15 cells. Often terminal knob.	Uncommon
M. gypseum	Flat, powdery-granular, central umbo with irregular fringe	White/cinnamon brown	Pale yellow–tan	Abundant ellipsoid shaped round tip, relatively thin spinous walls contain 4–6 cells. No terminal knob.	Abundant
T. mentagrophytes (zoophilic form)	Flat, powdery	Cream–light buff	Yellow–buff tan occasionally dark red/brown	Rare structures, cigar shaped. Thin smooth walls.	Abundant
T. mentagrophytes var erinacei	Flat with raised centre, granular	White/cream	Brilliant yellow	Very rare, when present irregular shape and size, thin smooth walls, contain 2–6 cells.	Abundant
M. persicolor	Folded granular, fringed periphery	Light buff	Peach-rose/deep ochre	Sparse, elongate, thin smooth walls with spinous tips, on short stalk. Multi-cellular.	Abundant

Systemic treatment

- Indications – generalised dermatophytosis and any local lesions unresponsive after 3–4 weeks of topical treatment.
- In kittens less than 12 weeks old, systemic therapy should be avoided if possible.
- All of the systemic drugs for dermatophytosis are potentially teratogenic.
- Initial therapy using Griseofulvin (Grisovin, Schering–Plough)
  - 25–60 mg/kg once or twice daily in oil.
  - Can cause bone marrow suppression.
  - White blood cell counts can be performed every 2 weeks to monitor bone marrow.
  - A marked clinical improvement should be seen within 6–8 weeks.
  - If no improvement:
    Check diagnosis.
    Check for immunosuppressive factors.
    Switch to itraconazole.
- Itraconazole (Sporonox, Janssen)
  - 10 mg/kg daily or alternate days.
  - As good or better than griseofulvin.
  - Well tolerated in cats.
  - Side effects rare.
  - Expensive.
- (Ketoconazole (Nizoral, Janssen) not recommended for therapy in cats. Less effective than griseofulvin. Hepatotoxic. 25% of cats exhibit side effects.)
- Providing improvement is seen, reculture after 6–8 weeks and then every 2 weeks until three negative cultures have been obtained 2 weeks apart.
- Treatment course.
  - 6–20 weeks generalised dermatophytosis.
  - 6–12 months onychomycosis.

Treatment of pseudomycetoma

- Recurrence is common after any form of therapy.
- Surgical excision with wide margins gives highest success rate.
- Medical therapy up to 18 months with griseofulvin, itraconazole.

Environmental treatment, including fomites

- Vacuuming – floors, furniture, curtains, ideally daily.
- Destroy as many rugs, brushes, etc. as possible.
- Where furnishings cannot be destroyed use:
  - Liquid disinfection – sodium hypochlorite (1:10 dilution household bleach), or enilconazole on surfaces where possible.
  - Fogging – enilconazole foggers.

Dermatophyte vaccines

- Limited availability in Europe.
- Useful to aid in treatment and prevention, as part of a total programme.

Cattery management of dermatophytosis

General points

This is an expensive procedure if performed adequately. Costing should be based on:

- Loss of revenue through cessation of breeding programme and selling of cats/kittens.
- Systemic drug therapy for all cats over the age of 12 weeks (except pregnant individuals which cannot be treated until after kitttening) for up to 16–20 weeks for short haired cats, more in long haired.
- Topical therapy and/or clipping.
- Routine ectoparasitic control.
- Laboratory tests:
  ○ Multiple fungal culture, initially to assess degree of cattery contamination and then three per cat before cessation of therapy.
  ○ Routine monitoring to assess bone marrow suppression (optional at the discretion of vet and owner).
- Treatment of the environment with liquid disinfectants/foggers.

Options for therapy

- Aim for complete eradication of dermatophytes from the cattery (Protocol 1).
- Depopulation of the cattery (Protocol 2).
- Treatment of only those cats leaving the premise (Protocol 3).

Protocol 1. Complete eradication of dermatophytes from the cattery

- Assessment of degree of infection.
  ○ Toothbrush cultures performed on all cats.
  ○ Toothbrush cultures from environment, especially from soft furnishings, window ledges, heating vents.
- Close the cattery to all visitors, stop breeding programmes, sale of kittens, etc.
- Isolate all cats that are culture negative in a culture negative environment (Group 1).
- Isolate all pregnant queens (Group 2).
- Isolate all breeding males (Group 3). Two separate groups, e.g. Group 3a (negative culture) and Group 3b (positive culture) can be created if necessary.

- Isolate all other positive cats (Group 4).
- Prevent cross contamination to non-infected groups. All grooming equipment, feeding bowls, utensils, etc., should be confined to each group. Where possible specific persons should be allocated to the care of each group.
- All cats should have routine ectoparasitic control used on them throughout the treatment period.

Group 1

- Weekly topical treatment with an antifungal rinse or shampoo.
- Where cats develop lesions these should be cultured and positive cats transferred to Group 4.
- Samples from all cats and their environment in this group should be taken by the toothbrush technique and cultured once treatment of other groups is completed and before mixing is allowed.

Group 2

- Queens – topical therapy with an antifungal rinse or shampoo until kittening, then as Group 4.
- Kittens – topical therapy until at least 12 weeks of age when systemic therapy can be started as Group 4.

Group 3

- Positive cultures as Group 4.
- Negative cultures as Group 1.

Group 4

- Treatment of cats.
  - All cats treated with topical therapy with an antifungal rinse or shampoo every 3–7 days, in addition to systemic therapy.
  - Clipping may be performed.
  - Initial drug of choice griseofulvin, given until all clinical lesions have resolved.
  - Toothbrush cultures should then be performed.
  - Treatment can be discontinued when three negative cultures have been obtained.
  - Negative cats can be moved to Group 1.
- Environmental decontamination.
  - Thorough cleaning including vacuuming to remove infected material.
  - Liquid disinfection of all available surfaces.
  - Enilconazole foggers can be used to treat bedding, etc., that can not be soaked or discarded.

Protocol 2. Depopulation of the cattery

- Rehoming or euthanasia (at owner's request) of all infected animals.
- Thorough decontamination of environment (liquid disinfection/foggers).
- Repopulation after three negative cultures from the environment 2 weeks apart.

Protocol 3. Treatment of only those cats leaving the premises

- No attempt is made to treat any cats in the cattery, which is accepted as having endemic ringworm.
- Isolation facilities should be made available for outgoing cats and kittens. The isolation facility allows any cat to be separated and treated with systemic and topical therapy to resolve the dermatophytosis before leaving the cattery.
- Pregnant queens can be started on a chlorhexidine-based product, used once or twice weekly, during pregnancy, e.g. Malaseb (Leo Labs). When kittens are born start the queen on griseofulvin.
- At 4 weeks of age culture samples from the kittens and begin topical therapy as queens.
    - Any positive kittens can be started on griseofulvin at 12 weeks.
    - Griseofulvin has been used in kittens as young as 6 weeks without ill effects.
    - The potential for side effects in this age of cat should be explained to the owner before use.
- No cat should leave the cattery until three negative cultures have been obtained 2 weeks apart.
- This can be used for queens wishing to go out to stud and for kittens to be sold.
- Queens must be clear of all therapy before mating.

Chapter 4

Other Fungal Skin Diseases

- A mycosis (plural mycoses) is a disease caused by a fungus.
- Mycoses can be classified according to their depth of infection as:
  - ○ Superficial.
  - ○ Subcutaneous (intermediate).
  - ○ Systemic (deep).

SUPERFICIAL MYCOSES

- Fungal infections of the superficial layers of skin, hairs and claws.
  - ○ Dermatophytosis.
  - ○ Candidiasis.
  - ○ Malasseziasis.
  - ○ Rhodotorulosis.

Dermatophytosis

See Chapter 3.

Candidiasis

Cause and pathogenesis

- Very rare disease in the cat – caused by *Candida* sp.
- Opportunistic infection caused by loss of integrity of skin and mucocutaneous areas, due to, e.g. trauma, burns.

Predisposing factors

- Immunosuppression through:
  - ○ Disease, e.g. viral infection (FIV, FeLV), neoplasia.
  - ○ Drug therapy, e.g. glucocorticoids.

Clinical signs

- Lesions found at moist macerated areas of skin and mucous membranes, e.g. intertriginous areas, mucocutaneous junctions, paws.
- Skin – oozing erythematous plaques and ulcers.

Differential diagnosis

Skin

- Eosinophilic granuloma complex.
- Dermatophytosis.
- Pemphigus foliaceus.
- Drug eruptions.

Diagnosis

- Clinical signs.
- Cytology – smear or acetate tape, typical budding yeasts.
- Culture – Sabouraud's dextrose agar.
- Biopsy.

Treatment

- Correction of underlying factors essential.

Local lesions

- Clipping and application of topical treatment three times daily.
- Suitable products contain nystatin, miconazole, clotrimazole, potassium permanganate.

Generalised lesions

- Systemic treatment itraconazole – 5–10 mg/kg every 24–48 hours.

Malasseziasis

Cause and pathogenesis

- Caused by skin commensal *Malassezia pachydermatis*.
- Rare reports have implicated *M. sympodialis* and *M. globosa* (lipid dependent yeasts) in some cases.
- Invasion of superficial epidermal layers occurs due to changes in surface microclimate by:
  - Increased sebum/cerumen production.
  - Moist maceration of skin.
  - Trauma.

Predisposing factors

- Allergy.
- Endocrine disease – especially hyperthyroidism (Fig. 4.1).
- Neoplasia, e.g. thymoma.
- Internal disease – especially those affecting lipid metabolism (Fig. 4.2).
- Therapy for the above – especially glucocorticoids in allergy (Fig. 4.3).

Clinical signs

- No age or sex incidence.
- Predisposed breeds – Devon Rex.
- Pruritus variable.
- Generalised lesions
  - ○ Malodorous erythematous dermatitis.
- Localised lesions.
  - ○ Black ceruminous otitis externa.
  - ○ Thick greasy exudation associated with chin acne, 'stud tail', interdigital dermatitis.

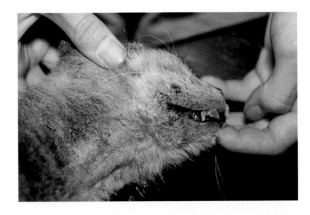

Fig. 4.1 *Malassezia* secondary to hyperthyroidism.

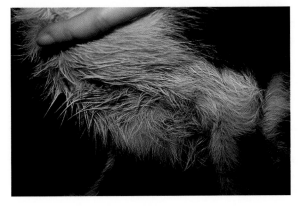

Fig. 4.2 *Malassezia* secondary to hepatic carcinoma.

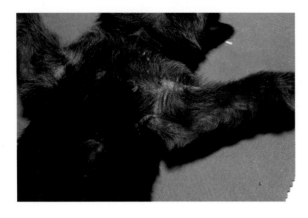

Fig. 4.3 *Malassezia* in elbow flexures secondary to steroid therapy in an atopic cat.

Differential diagnosis

- Allergy (food, atopy, fleas).
- Demodicosis.
- Neoplasia (epitheliotrophic lymphoma).
- Hyperthyroidism.

These diseases can occur concurrently with *Malassezia* dermatitis.

Diagnosis

- Clinical signs.
- Cytology of skin scrapings, direct smears, acetate tape impression smears stained with Diff Quik – typical budding yeasts (dark blue/purple peanut shaped organisms).
- Culture – contact plates (lipid-dependent species require special mycological media).
- Biopsy.

Treatment

- Therapy of predisposing factors is essential.
- When predisposing factors cannot be identified or treated adequately, chronic therapy is indicated.
- No veterinary products are licensed to treat this disease in the cat.

Topical treatment

- Applied twice weekly to localised or generalised disease until a clinical improvement is seen, then reduced to every 10–14 days for maintenance.
- Shampoo – miconazole/chlorhexidine (Malaseb, Leo Laboratories), selenium sulphide (Seleen, Sanofi) followed by enilconazole rinse (Imaverol, Janssen).
- Creams/lotion containing miconazole, enilconazole.

Systemic treatment

- Itraconazole (Sporonox, Janssen) – 5mg/kg once daily.

Rhodotorulosis

Cause and pathogenesis

- Very rare disease caused by skin commensal *Rhodotorula* spp.
- Commensal organisms can cause disease as opportunistic pathogens in immunosuppressed cats (Fig. 4.4).

Predisposing factors

- Immunosuppression due to viral disease, e.g. FeLV, FIV.

Clinical signs

- Generalised erythematous dermatitis, brown/red crusting at mucocutaneous junctions.

Differential diagnosis

- As malasseziasis.

Diagnosis

- Clinical signs.
- Culture.
- Biopsy.

Treatment

- Treatment of underlying immunosuppression where possible, then as malasseziasis.

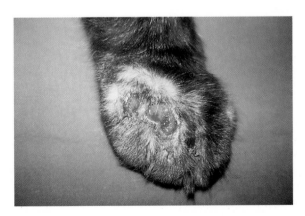

Fig. 4.4 Skin disease caused by opportunistic fungus *Exophilia weneckii* (picture courtesy R. Bond).

SUBCUTANEOUS MYCOSES (INTERMEDIATE MYCOSES)

- Fungal infections of viable skin, usually caused by infection of traumatised skin by saprophytes.
  - Eumycotic mycetoma.
  - Phaeohyphomycosis.
  - Zygomycosis.
  - Sporotrichosis.

Eumycotic mycetoma

Cause and pathogenesis

- Rare disease in Europe and USA caused by wound contamination by soil saprophytes especially *Pseudoallescheria boydii*.

Clinical signs

- Lesions usually solitary nodules – especially on extremities.
- Triad of signs.
  - Nodular swelling.
  - Draining fistulas (discharge variable colour).
  - Granules.
- Dematiaceous fungi – black grained mycetoma, e.g. *Curvularia geniculata*.
- Non-pigmented fungi – white grained mycetoma, e.g. *Pseudoallescheria boydii*.
- Chronic infections can extend into underlying bone or muscle.

Differential diagnosis

- Cat bite abscesses.
- Eosinophilic granuloma complex.
- Infectious granulomas, e.g. bacteria, fungi.
- Foreign body granuloma.
- Neoplasia.
- Plasma cell pododermatitis.

Diagnosis

- Clinical signs.
- Cytology of aspirates, direct smears or squashed preparations of grains reveal fungi.
- Culture of grains or biopsy material on Sabouraud's dextrose agar.
- Biopsy – fungal elements as grains.

Treatment

- Wide surgical incision; often amputation of limb is necessary.
- Medical therapy – poor response: possible itraconazole – 5–10 mg/kg daily up to 2–3 months beyond clinical cure.

Phaeohyphomycosis

Cause and pathogenesis

- Uncommon disease caused by wound contamination by saprophytic fungi found in soil and organic materials.
- No granules, but fungi form pigmented hyphae.

Clinical signs

- Solitary slow growing subcutaneous nodules.
- Especially affecting paw, leg, nose or trunk.
- Lesions may ulcerate and develop draining tracts.
- Systemic spread unusual.

Differential diagnosis

- As eumycotic mycetoma.

Diagnosis

- Clinical signs.
- Cytology of aspirate or direct smear – pigmented fungi may be seen.
- Culture preferably of biopsy material on Sabouraud's dextrose agar.
- Biopsy.

Treatment

- Wide surgical excision – recurrence common.
- Chemotherapy – response unpredictable.
- Possible itraconazole ± flucytosine, or amphotericin B ± flucytosine.

Zygomycosis

- Two orders can cause this disease:
  - Mucorales, e.g. *Rhizopus* spp.
  - Entomophthorales, e.g. *Conidobolus* spp.

Cause and pathogenesis

- Rare disease caused by ubiquitous soil saprophytes.
- Organisms also found as flora of skin and hair coat.
- Produce infection through wound contamination.

Predisposing factors

• Immunosuppression may be important in some cases.

Clinical signs

• Usually causes fatal gastrointestinal disease.
• Cutaneous lesions – solitary or multiple ulcerated draining nodules, especially extremities.

Differential diagnosis

• As eumycotic mycetoma.

Diagnosis

• Clinical signs.
• Cytology of aspirate or direct smear – fungal elements present.
• Culture of biopsy material on Sabouraud's dextrose agar.
• Biopsy – fungal elements visible.

Treatment

• Surgical excision where possible or debulking therapy plus chemotherapy with amphotericin B or itraconazole.

Sporotrichosis

Cause and pathogenesis

• An uncommon disease caused by ubiquitous soil saprophyte *Sporothrix schenckii*.
• Infection caused by inoculation of organism by contaminated teeth or claw from other cats during fights.
• Zoonotic disease.

Clinical signs

• Breed predisposition – Siamese.
• Sex predisposition – entire male cats due to fighting.
• Age predisposition – young cats < 4 years.

Cutaneous form

• Multiple ulcerated nodules and plaques especially on head, pinnae and trunk; no systemic signs.
• Initial signs may be of fight wound abscess.
• Skin necrosis may occur to reveal underlying muscle or bone.
• Normal grooming can spread infection to other areas by autoinoculation.

Cutaneolymphatic form

- Single nodule on limb leads to ascending lymphatic infection – regional lymphadenopathy.

Disseminated form

- Infection can spread to internal organs, especially if cats are given glucocorticoids.
- Cats often present with lethargy, depression, anorexia and pyrexia.

Differential diagnosis

- As eumycotic mycetoma.

Diagnosis

- Care should be taken when handling infected cats. Organisms are found in tissue, exudates and faeces. High risk of human contagion.
- Clinical signs.
- Cytology of aspirate or direct smear – organisms numerous and appear as typical round, oval or cigar shaped.
- Culture of both exudate and biopsy sample on Sabouraud's dextrose agar.
- Biopsy – fungal elements numerous.

Treatment

- Potassium iodide – oral administration of saturated solution at 20 mg/kg once or twice daily for 30 days beyond clinical cure.
  - Iodism common side effects leading to withdrawal of therapy – vomiting, anorexia, neurological signs, cardiovascular effects.
- Itraconazole – 5–10 mg/kg every 24–48 hours.
- Approximately 50% of cases respond to medical therapy.
- Glucocorticoids are contraindicated in all cases. Even after apparent cure these can cause recurrence.

SYSTEMIC MYCOSES

- Fungal infections of internal organs caused by soil saprophytes.
  - Blastomycosis
  - Coccidiodomycosis
  - Cryptococcosis
  - Histoplasmosis
  - Prototothecosis
- Contagion usually occurs by inhalation, direct cutaneous inoculation is rare – usually haematogenous spread to skin.

- Infection can be associated with immunosuppression due to:
  - Viral infection with FIV, FeLV.
  - Glucocorticoid administration.

Blastomycosis

Cause and pathogenesis

- Very rare disease caused by *Blastomyces dermatitidis* – especially seen in areas with sandy soil close to water.
- Zoonotic disease – can be spread by bites from infected cats.

Clinical signs

- Breed predisposition – Abyssinian, Havana brown, Siamese.
- Sex predisposition – entire male cats due to fighting.
- Age predisposition – none.
- Systemic signs – disseminated disease is common:
  - ~60% respiratory signs.
  - ~55% weight loss.
  - ~40% neurological signs.
- Only ~25% of cases have skin disease variable. Lesions range from single draining nodules to widespread cellulitis, especially affecting digits and face.

Diagnosis

Skin disease

- Clinical signs.
- Cytology of aspirates or direct smear – oval broad based budding yeast with thick cell walls.
- Culture not recommended.
- Biopsy – fungal elements easily seen.

Treatment

- Poor prognosis as many have disseminated disease.
- Isolated cutaneous lesions can be surgically removed (with care due to risk of contagion).
- Combination of itraconazole sequentially with amphotericin B.

Coccidiodomycosis

Cause and pathogenesis

- Very rare disease caused by *Coccidioides immitis* – especially seen in areas with sandy, alkaline soils.
- Zoonotic disease.

Clinical signs

- Breed, sex and age predisposition – none.
- Systemic signs – disseminated disease is common.
  - ~25% respiratory signs.
  - ~45% weight loss.
  - Musculoskeletal and neurological signs in <20%.
- Cutaneous lesions – approximately 56% of cases have multiple ulcerated nodules.

Diagnosis

Skin lesions

- Clinical signs.
- Cytology of aspirates or direct smears – fungal elements rarely seen.
- Culture not recommended.
- Biopsy – uncommon fungal elements seen as large spherules containing numerous endospores.
- Agar gel immunodiffusion.

Treatment

- Moderate response to medical therapy – approximately 66% response.
- Itraconazole – up to 1 year of treatment usually required.

Cryptococcosis

Cause and pathogenesis

- Uncommon disease caused by *Cryptococcus neoformans* – especially associated with pigeon droppings.
- Immunosuppressed animals susceptible.

Clinical signs

- Breed predisposition – Abyssinian, Siamese.
- Systemic signs – disseminated disease is common.
  - ~65% nasal discharge.
  - Neurological, ocular and gastrointestinal signs also common.
- Cutaneous lesions.
  - 70% of cats with nasal discharge have associated intranasal polyp or granuloma on the bridge of the nose (Figs 4.5, 4.6).
  - 40% of affected cats have primary skin involvement presenting as multiple nodules, abscesses, especially on face, pinnae and paws.

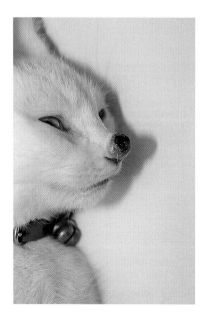

Fig. 4.5 Ulcerated granuloma on the bridge of the nose in a cat with cryptococcosis.

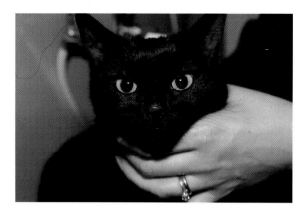

Fig. 4.6 Hyperpigmented granuloma on nose caused by cryptococcosis.

Diagnosis

Skin lesions

- Clinical signs – especially nasal signs.
- Cytology of aspirates or direct smear – numerous round/elliptical yeast-like organisms, narrow-based buds with capsule (appear as clear halo).
- Culture not recommended.
- Biopsy – special stains of capsules.
- Serology – latex agglutination test.

Treatment

- Solitary lesions can be surgically removed.
- Generalised disease chemotherapy – itraconazole can be combined with flucytosine.
- Glucocorticoids contraindicated.

Histoplasmosis

Cause and pathogenesis

- Rare disease caused by *Histoplasma capsulatum* – especially moist humid environments often associated with birds and bat droppings.

Clinical signs

- Breed predisposition – Siamese.
- Systemic disease – disseminated disease common.
  - ~40% respiratory signs.
  - ~65% pyrexia.
  - Gastrointestinal, ocular signs less common.
- Cutaneous lesions are less common than systemic signs and appear as multiple, ulcerated papules and nodules at any site.

Diagnosis

Skin lesions

- Clinical signs.
- Cytology of aspirate or direct smear – numerous small round yeast-like bodies with narrow halo.
- Culture not recommended.
- Biopsy – numerous intracellular organisms.
- Serology – not reliable.

Treatment

- Very poor prognosis.
- Itraconazole most useful. In severe cases it can be used in combination with amphotericin B.
- Treatment may be needed for life.

Protothecosis

Cause and pathogenesis

- Rare disease caused by *Prototheca* sp. especially *Prototheca wickerhamii*.
- Saprophytic algae found in sewage and stagnant water.

Table 4.1 Systemic anti-fungal therapy

Drug	Dose rate	Indication
Amphotericin B	0.5 mg/kg alternate day i.v. in 5% dextrose and water	Systemic mycoses, *Blastomyces, Histoplasma, Cryptococcus* (usually in combination with itraconazole)
Flucytosine	25–35 mg/kg p.o. every 8 hours	*Cryptococcus, Phaehyphomycosis*
Griseofulvin	20–60 mg/kg p.o. twice daily in oil	Dermatophytes
Itraconazole	5–10 mg/kg p.o. once daily	Dermatophytes, *Candida, Malassezia, Aspergillus,* subcutaneous and deep mycoses (often with amphotericin B)
Potassium iodide	20 mg/kg p.o. once or twice daily with food	Sporotrichosis

Key: p.o., by mouth; i.v., intravenous.

- Opportunistic invader of contaminated wounds.
- Disseminated disease associated with immunosuppression.

Clinical signs

- Systemic disease – not reported in the cat.
- Cutaneous lesions – solitary or multiple papules, nodules or subcutaneous growths.
- Lesions most commonly on paws and legs. Also around head and tail base.

Diagnosis

Skin lesions

- Clinical signs.
- Cytology of aspirates or direct smears – numerous intercellular spherules containing endospores.
- Culture of biopsy material on Sabouraud's dextrose agar or blood agar.
- Biopsy – numerous fungal elements present.
- Fluorescent antibody technique on formal fixed tissue.

Treatment

- Surgical excision of cutaneous lesions where possible.
- Chemotherapy – 3–4 weeks beyond clinical cure. Amphotericin B with itraconazole.

Chapter 5

Parasitic Skin Diseases

ARTHROPOD PARASITES

ARACHNIDS

MITES

- *Otodectes cynotis.*
- Cheyletiellosis.
- Demodicosis.
- Feline scabies.
- Trombiculiasis.
- *Dermanyssus gallinae.*
- *Lynxacarus radovsky.*

Otodectes cynotis

Cause and pathogenesis

- Psoroptiform mite – non-burrowing, lives and feeds on the surface of the skin, especially in the ears.
- Highly contagious – passed from dam to kittens and kitten to kitten.

Clinical signs

- Otitis externa.
  - Cerumenous discharge from ear canal – 'coffee ground' appearance (Fig. 5.1).
  - Symptoms variable from heavy discharge–minimal pruritus to minimal discharge–severe pruritus (Fig. 5.2).
- Ectopic infestation – mites move out of ear especially when cat curled up.
  - Can spread to neck, rump and tail.
  - Can be asymptomatic or pruritic.
  - Lesions can mimic those of miliary dermatitis, ventral or flank alopecia.

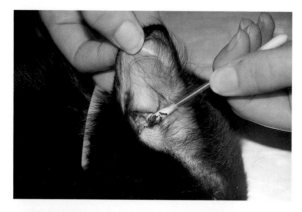

Fig. 5.1 'Coffee ground' discharge typical of *Otodectes cynotis*.

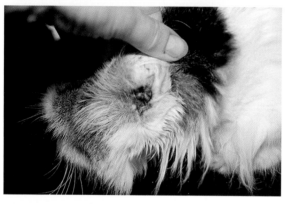

Fig. 5.2 Aural discharge with only mild pruritus in *Otodectes* infestation.

Differential diagnosis

- Otitis externa.
  - ○ Allergic otitis.
  - ○ Demodicosis.
  - ○ Dermatophytosis.
- Ectopic infestation.
  - ○ Flea allergic dermatitis.
  - ○ Other allergies (atopy, food 'allergy').
  - ○ Ectoparasites (*Cheyletiella*, lice, *Trombicula*).
  - ○ Dermatophytosis.
  - ○ Other differentials of miliary dermatitis (see Chapter 17).
  - ○ Other differentials of ventral or flank alopecia (see Chapter 9).

Distinguishing features

- See Figs 5.3 (adult) and 5.4 (eggs).
- Oval mite, four pairs of legs; all except rudimentary fourth pair of female extend beyond body margin.
- Male – all legs short unjointed pedicles with suckers.
- Female – first two pairs of legs have pedicles with suckers.
- Terminal anus.

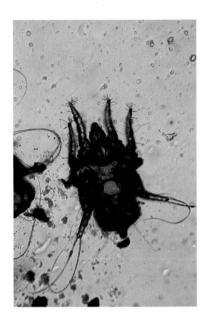

Fig. 5.3 *Otodectes cynotis* mite.

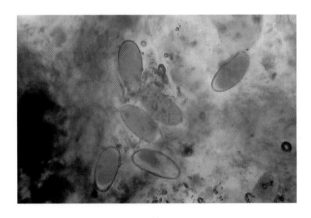

Fig. 5.4 *Otodectes cynotis* eggs.

Life cycle – host specific

MALE ADULTS   EGGS   4-day incubation

         ADULTS   LARVAE (6 legs)

                            21 days   3–12 days feed/rest

Copulate if
females develop

DEUTONYMPHS (8 legs)   PROTONYMPHS (8 legs)

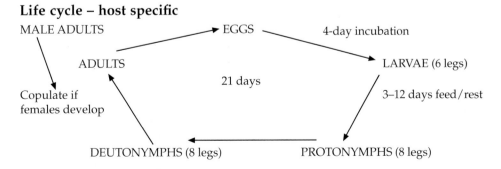

- Can exist in the environment for short periods.

Diagnosis

- Clinical signs.
- Identification of mites in ear wax microscopically.
- Ectopic infestation – skin scrapings or acetate tapes.

Treatment

- Miticidal therapy should be applied to the ear and the body in all cases.
- Topical therapy – use a combination of:
  - ○ Aural miticidal drops – Auroto (Arnolds), Canaural (Leo Labs), Oterna (Schering Plough), GAC (Arnolds). Use at manufacturer's suggested interval for a minimum of 28 days with
  - ○ Insecticidal powders/sprays for body.
- Alternatively, ivermectin (unlicensed for use in cats) may be used in wild cats and difficult cases in catteries – 200–400 μg/kg by mouth or subcutaneous injection at 10 daily intervals on three occasions. Will replace body and otic treatment.
- Anti-inflammatories – prednisolone – 1 mg/kg for 7–10 days.

Cheyletiellosis

Cause and pathogenesis

- Common disease caused by *Cheyletiella* spp.
- Non-burrowing surface living and feeding parasite leads to typical 'walking dandruff'.
- Zoonosis – human lesions – pruritic papules at contact sites with animal.
- Large mites – although *C. blakei* is recognised as the species found on cats, *C. yasguri* (dog species) and *C. parasitovorax* (rabbit species) can also be isolated.
- Highly contagious.

Clinical signs

- Young and immunosuppressed animals predisposed.
- Variable presentation can be asymptomatic.
- Often a pruritic cat will overgroom and remove much of the scaling.
- Usually dorsal scaling with increased degree of pruritus leading to self-inflicted trauma.
- Can present as miliary dermatitis, eosinophilic granulomas, or ventral or flank alopecia (Fig. 5.5).

Differential diagnosis

- As ectopic *Otodectes*.

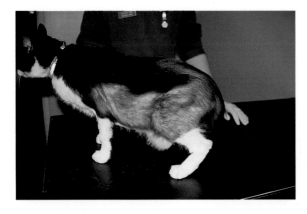

Fig. 5.5 Flank alopecia secondary to *Cheyletiella*.

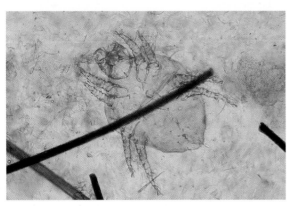

Fig. 5.6 *Cheyletiella* mite.

Distinguishing features

- Large mite saddle shaped (Fig. 5.6).
- Four pairs of legs bear combs.
- Accessory mouth parts terminate in hooks (Fig. 5.7).
- Sensory organ on genu 1.
  - ○ Comb shape in *C. blakei*.
  - ○ Global shape in *C. parasitovorax*.
  - ○ Heart shape in *C. yasguri*.
- Egg attached to hair at one end only by filaments.

Life cycle – host specific

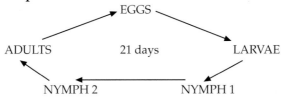

- Can live for a short period in the environment – females up to 10 days.

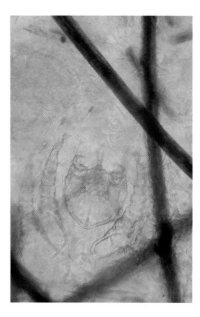

Fig. 5.7 Close up of *Cheyletiella* head showing hooks on accessory mouth parts.

Diagnosis

- Clinical signs.
- Identification of parasite – skin samples are best taken from areas relatively inaccessible to grooming activity of the cat, e.g. back of neck.
  - Coat brushing – direct examination with magnifying glass.
  - Superficial skin scrapings into mineral oil or potassium hydroxide (10%).
  - Acetate tape impression smears examined microscopically.
  - Faecal examination for *Cheyletiella* mites and eggs.
- Therapeutic trial.

Treatment

- Treatment of all in contact animals as well as those showing clinical signs.
- Treatment of animal.
  - Antiparasitic shampoo – selenium sulphide 1% (Seleen, Sanofi). Three treatments given at 10 day intervals.
  - Antiparasitic sprays – fipronil (Merial) may need to be used every 2–3 weeks (extra-label indication).
  - Antiparasitic spot-ons – limited efficacy.
  - Ivermectin (unlicensed for use in cats) – dosage 200–400 µg/kg by mouth or subcutaneous injection. Given at 10 daily intervals on three occasions.
- Environmental treatment insecticidal sprays:
  - Permethrin/cyromazine (Staykil, Novartis).
  - Pyrethrin/methoprene (Vet Kem Acclaim, Sanofi).

Demodicosis

Cause and pathogenesis

- Rare skin disease of cats caused by increased number of *Demodex* mites.
- Normal skin commensal recognised as:
  - ○ Follicular living mites – *Demodex cati* causes follicular demodicosis.
  - ○ Surface living short mites inhabit stratum corneum – *Demodex gatoi* causes superficial demodicosis.
  - ○ Third form of *Demodex* also thought to exist.
- Generalised demodicosis usually associated with underlying disease.
  - ○ Viral infection FIV, FeLV.
  - ○ Endocrine disease – diabetes mellitus, hyperadrenocorticism.
  - ○ Immune mediated disease – systemic lupus erythematosus.
  - ○ Steroid therapy.
- Predisposed breeds – Siamese and Burmese cats.

Clinical signs

Follicular demodicosis

- Pruritus is variable in both forms of the disease.
  - ○ Localised form:
    Patchy alopecia with erythema and scale.
    Affects face and head especially eyelids and periocular skin.
    Can occur as ceruminous otitis externa.
  - ○ Generalised form:
    Lesions – macules, alopecic patches (Fig. 5.8), hyperpigmentation, erythema and scaling.
    Affects head, also neck, trunk and limbs.

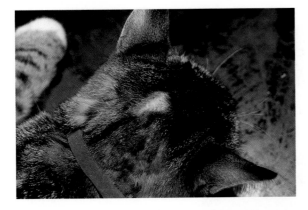

Fig. 5.8 Alopecic patch of follicular demodicosis caused by *Demodex cati*.

Superficial demodicosis

- Highly pruritic disease.
- Alopecia, crusting and excoriation due to severe self-inflicted trauma.
- Lesions usually concentrated on head, neck and elbows.
- Can present as non-scaling symmetric alopecia (Fig. 5.9).

Differential diagnosis

- Follicular demodicosis.
  - ○ Dermatophytosis.
  - ○ Ectoparasitic diseases – especially *Otodectes*.
  - ○ Cutaneous neoplasia.
  - ○ Primary ocular disease (localised form).
- Superficial demodicosis.
  - ○ Allergy (atopy, food 'allergy').
  - ○ Scabies.
  - ○ Flea allergic dermatitis.

Distinguishing features

- *Demodex cati* long cigar shaped mite.
- *Demodex gatoi* (Fig. 5.10) short blunt rounded abdomen.
- Both form adults and nymphs which have eight legs; larvae have six legs.
- Eggs slim oval shape.

Life cycle – host specific

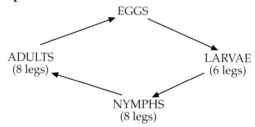

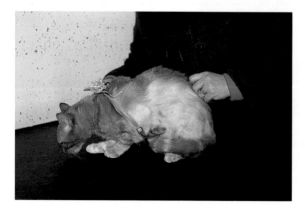

Fig. 5.9 Non-scaling symmetrical alopecia caused by *Demodex gatoi* (picture courtesy of J. Henfrey).

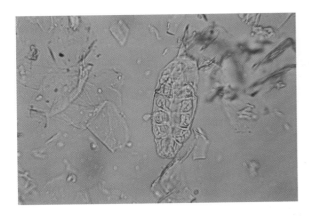

Fig. 5.10 Short non-follicular demodex *Demodex gatoi* (picture courtesy of A. Foster).

Diagnosis

- Skin scrapings.
  - Deep scrapings from areas of comedones.
  - Squeeze skin to extrude mites from follicles before scraping.
- Acetate tape impression smears.
  - Useful to identify superficial non-follicular mites.
- Histopathology.

Treatment

- No drug is licensed for treatment of demodectic mange in the cat.
- Some cats will respond in a short time with mild topical therapy.
- Clinical response is also dependent on immune status of the cat.
- Superficial mite treated more easily due to location in the skin.
  - Amitraz (Aludex, Hoechst) – 0.0125% solution, i.e. 0.25 ml of Aludex in 100 ml of water, applied weekly.
  - Selenium sulphide 1% (Seleen, Sanofi Animal Health) – used once weekly.
  - Ivermectin (Ivomec, Merial) – administered orally at 0.4 mg/kg daily (weeks to months). Dose should be started at 0.1 mg/kg daily and increased to 0.4 mg/kg over 5 days.

Feline scabies (notoedric mange)

- Highly contagious ectoparasitic disease caused by *Notoedres cati.*
- Mite belongs to family Sarcoptidae; life cycle is similar to *Sarcoptes scabiei.*
- Zoonosis – human lesions papular eruptions on arms and trunk; self-limiting unless there is repeated contact with infected animals.
- Very rare disease in the UK.
- *Sarcoptes scabiei* var. *canis* can also be rarely seen in cats. Clinical findings are similar to those described for notoedric mange (Fig. 5.11).

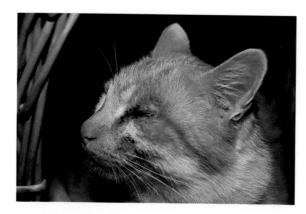

Fig. 5.11 Self-inflicted trauma to the face due to *Sarcoptes scabiei*.

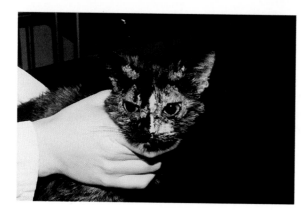

Fig. 5.12 Facial excoriation due to *Notoedres cati* (picture courtesy of J. Henfrey).

Cause and pathogenesis

- *N. cati* primarily infests cats but can also affect foxes, dogs and rabbits.
- An obligate parasite, it survives off-host only a few days.
- Infested cats carry large numbers of mites, easily found on scrapings.

Clinical signs

- Lesions initially found on edge of ear pinna, spread rapidly to rest of face and neck (Fig. 5.12).
- Cat's grooming activities lead to further spread to feet and perineum.
- Pruritus poorly controlled with glucocorticoids.
- Skin thickened and covered with thick yellow/grey crusts with papules.
- Self-inflicted trauma leads to excoriation.
- Chronic disease will generalise.

Differential diagnosis

- Allergy (atopy, food).
- Cheyletiellosis.

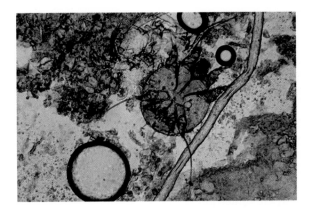

Fig. 5.13 *Sarcoptes scabiei* mite.

- *Otodectes cynotis.*
- Pediculosis.
- Pemphigus foliaceus.

Distinguishing features of *Notoedres cati* compared to *Sarcoptes scabiei* (Fig. 5.13).

- Oval mite, eggs round (smaller than *Sarcoptes*).
- Two pairs anterior legs, long medium length, unjointed stalks with suckers.
- Two pairs posterior legs do not extend beyond the borders of the body.
- Body shows obvious striations.
- Dorsal anus (terminal anus *Sarcoptes*).

Life cycle

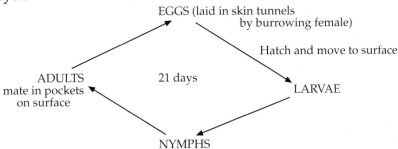

- Survival off the host, approximately 7 days.

Diagnosis

- History of non-seasonal pruritus that is poorly responsive to steroids.
- Clinical signs – especially presence of intense pruritus.
- Skin scrapings – deep scrapings. Mites easier to find than scabies mites, but are small and best identified under low power with reduced light.
- Biopsy – mites occasionally found.

- Therapeutic trial – improvement after treatment with miticide allows retrospective diagnosis.

Treatment

- Animal treatment – no licensed product available in UK for the treatment of cats.
  - Amitraz (Aludex, Hoechst) – 0.0125% solution, i.e. 0.25 ml of Aludex in 100 ml of water, applied weekly for four applications.
  - Ivermectin (Ivomec, Merial) – subcutaneously at 0.3 mg/kg weekly for four treatments.
- Environmental treatment.
  - Permethrin/cyromazine (Staykil, Novartis).
  - Pyrethrin/methoprene (Vet Kem Acclaim, Sanofi).
- Glucocorticoids – 7–10 days of prednisolone at 1.0–2.0 mg/kg each morning may be useful after a diagnosis has been made.

Trombiculiasis

- Seasonal pruritic skin disease caused commonly by harvest mite *Neotrombicula* (*Trombicula*) *autumnalis*, also *Walchia americana* in the USA.

Cause and pathogenesis

- Larval form is parasitic on animals.
- Seen in grassland in late summer/early autumn, especially on chalky soils.

Clinical signs

- Larvae usually in and around the ears (Fig. 5.14).
- Bright red dots 'paprika' in appearance.
- Papulocrustous eruptions caused by larvae feeding.

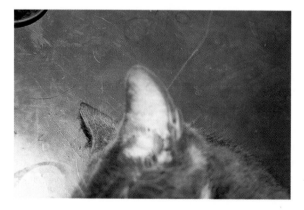

Fig. 5.14 Bright red *Trombicula* larvae on ear pinna.

Differential diagnosis

- Allergy (atopy, contact allergy).
- *Otodectes cynotis.*
- *Spilopsyllus cuniculi.*
- Pediculosis.

Distinguishing features

Larval form (Fig. 5.15) is parasitic – six legged, bright red in colour, size of pinhead.

Life cycle

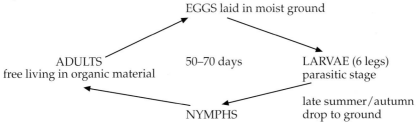

Diagnosis

- Larvae seen with naked eye as bright orange/red dots.
- Skin scrapings into mineral oil as mites are active and will escape.

Treatment

- Antiparasitic washes or sprays (see *Cheyletiella*).
- Glucocorticoids, e.g. prednisolone – 1.0–2.0 mg/kg daily for 2–3 days.

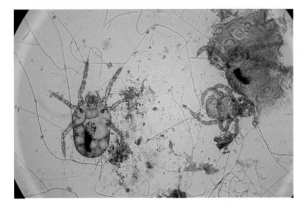

Fig. 5.15 *Trombicula autumnalis* larva.

Dermanyssus gallinae

- The poultry mite *Dermanyssus gallinae* causes a non-seasonal pruritic skin disease in cats.

Cause and pathogenesis

- Non-host specific ectoparasite will attack dogs, cats, man as well as birds.
- Adult mite lives in nests and cracks in poultry cages/houses.
- Animals are infected through environmental contamination.

Clinical signs

- Erythema, papulocrustous eruptions, especially dorsum and extremities.

Differential diagnosis

- As ectopic *Otodectes*.

Distinguishing features

- Eight legged white/grey/black mite up to 1.0 mm (Fig. 5.16).
- Red when engorged.
- First pair of appendages (chelicerae) whip-like.
- Anus posterior half of anal plate.

Life cycle

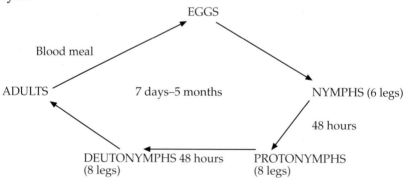

- Lives in the environment.

Diagnosis

- History of exposure to poultry.
- Typical red mites identified in scrapings.

Treatment

- Animal treatment as *Cheyletiella*.
- Environmental treatment.

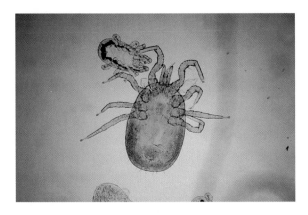

Fig. 5.16 *Dermanyssus gallinae* mite.

○ Permethrin/cyromazine (Staykil, Novartis).
○ Pyrethrin/methoprene (Vet Kem Acclaim, Sanofi).
○ *Dermanyssus gallinae* can show resistance to pyrethroids.

Lynxacarus radovsky

- Cat fur mite very rare in the UK.
- May be found on imported animals.

Cause and pathogenesis

- Small fur clasping mite.
- Poorly contagious – infections occur through direct contact or via fomites.
- Similar in appearance to other fur mites – identification requires a competent parasitologist.

Clinical signs

- Often asymptomatic, although coat appears dull.
- Mites usually attach to the ends of hairs on the dorsum to give the coat a 'salt-and-pepper' appearance.
- Damaged hair can be easily epilated.
- May present with signs of miliary dermatitis.

Differential diagnosis

- As ectopic *Otodectes*.

Distinguishing features

- Elongated body 430–520 μm in length.
- Flap-like sternal extensions contain first two grasping legs.
- All legs have terminal suckers.

Diagnosis

- Isolation of mites on skin scrapings or acetate tape impressions.

Treatment

- As *Cheyletiella*.

TICKS

- Argasid – soft ticks.
- Ixodid – hard ticks.

Argasid ticks

- Spinous ear tick – *Otobius megnini*.
- Found in warm climates.
- Causes acute otitis externa.

Ixodid ticks

Cause and pathogenesis

- Common ticks in the UK include *Ixodes ricinus* (caster bean tick), *Ixodes hexagonus* (hedgehog tick).
- Large parasites approximately 0.5 cm long.
- No breed, sex or age predilection.

Clinical signs

- Tick attaches to an area in contact with the ground (Fig. 5.17).
- Asymptomatic in some animals.

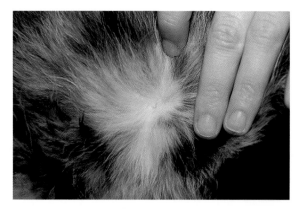

Fig. 5.17 *Ixodes ricinus* tick on the head.

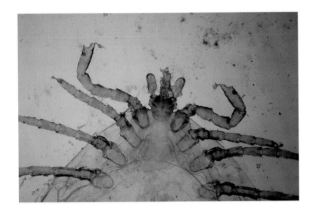

Fig. 5.18 Head of *Ixodes ricinus* tick.

- Local irritation/hypersensitivity can lead to lick granuloma formation.
- Ticks can be vectors of bacterial, rickettsial, viral and protozoal diseases.

Diagnosis

- Clinical signs.
- Identification of parasite (Fig. 5.18).

Life cycle

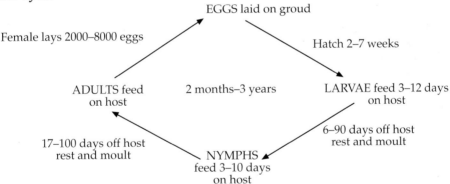

Treatment

Ticks

- Careful manual removal using spirit swab or mosquito forceps.
- Insecticidal spray – fipronil (Frontline, Merial), dichlorvos (Nuvan Top, Novartis).

Granuloma

- Surgical removal.

INSECTS

- Fleas
  - ○ Flea allergic dermatitis
- Lice
  - ○ Pediculosis
- Flies
  - ○ Mosquito dermatitis
  - ○ Fly dermatitis
  - ○ Myiasis
  - ○ Cuterebriasis
- Hymenoptera
  - ○ Stings

FLEAS

- The most common cause of skin disease in the cat.
- 97% of fleas found on cats are *Ctenocephalides felis felis*.
- Other species that may also be found on cats:
  - ○ *Ctenocephalides canis* (dog).
  - ○ *Spilopsyllus cuniculi* (rabbit).
  - ○ *Archaeopsylla erinacei* (hedgehog).

Flea allergic dermatitis

Cause and pathogenesis

- A very common pruritic skin disease of cats that have been sensitised to flea saliva.
- Can present in many different ways and should be considered as a differential diagnosis in almost any clinical presentation.
- Flea saliva contains at least 15 potentially allergenic components.
- These are complete antigens, not haptens.
- Non-allergic animals tolerate fleas and develop minimal clinical signs.
- In the cat the principal reaction is of a type I – immediate – hypersensitivity.
- A type IV – delayed – hypersensitivity has not been identified.

Clinical signs

- No age incidence.
- Can present with many different clinical signs including:
  - ○ Papulocrustous reaction especially on the dorsum – 'miliary dermatitis' (Fig. 5.19).
  - ○ Self-induced symmetrical alopecia on ventrum or flanks (Fig. 5.20).

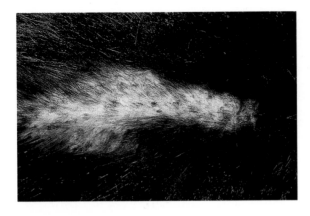

Fig. 5.19 Miliary dermatitis caused by flea allergic dermatitis.

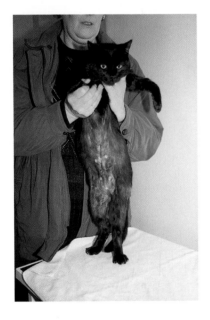

Fig. 5.20 Ventral abdominal alopecia caused by flea allergy.

- ○ Eosinophilic allergic syndrome (Fig. 5.21).
- ○ Facial pruritus.
- Many cats with flea allergic dermatitis have other allergies concurrently such as atopy and food intolerance.

Differential diagnosis

- Allergy especially food, atopy.
- Pediculosis.
- Cheyletiellosis.
- Ectopic *Otodectes*.
- Trombiculiasis.

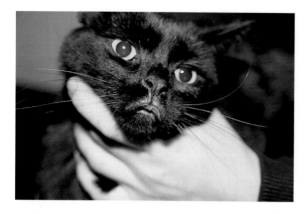

Fig. 5.21 Indolent ulcer secondary to flea allergic dermatitis.

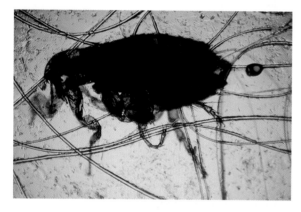

Fig. 5.22 Flea under acetate tape showing appearance of flea dirt under the microscope.

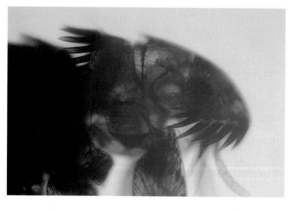

Fig. 5.23 Head of *Ctenocephalides felis* showing both genal and pronotal combs.

- Dermatophytosis.
- Psychogenic alopecia.

Distinguishing features

- Small brown wingless insects, body laterally compressed (Fig. 5.22).
- Elongated head.

- Both genal and pronotal combs present; eight or nine genal combs present; the first comb is the same length as the second (Fig. 5.23).

Life cycle

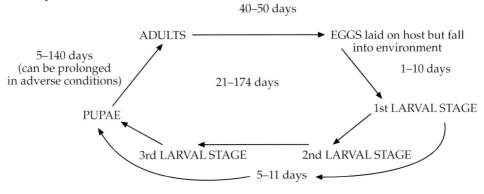

40–50 days

ADULTS ⟶ EGGS laid on host but fall into environment

5–140 days (can be prolonged in adverse conditions)

21–174 days

1–10 days

PUPAE

1st LARVAL STAGE

3rd LARVAL STAGE

2nd LARVAL STAGE

5–11 days

Diagnosis

- Clinical signs on cat and/or owner.
- Identification of fleas, flea 'dirt', flea eggs or *Dipylidium caninum* (the flea is the intermediate host for this tapeworm).
- Wet paper test – blood in flea faeces produces red streaks when coat is brushed onto wet paper (Fig. 5.24). This can be difficult to find due to cats' grooming activity.
- Acetate tape impressions from coat especially from inaccessible areas around the neck – microscopic examination reveals flea faeces.
- Histopathology – non-specific allergic reaction pattern.
- Intradermal testing with flea antigens (immediate reaction only).
- Response to flea control programme.
- Blood samples to look for Ig E to flea saliva (specialised laboratories).

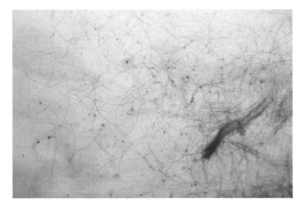

Fig. 5.24 Flea dirt on wet paper.

Treatment

Flea control

- This should be tailored to the individual based on numbers and types of pet, ability of owner to use particular products.
- Client education regarding flea life cycle is essential.
- Control of fleas in the environment.
  - ○ Internal environment most important in temperate climate.
  - ○ Thorough vacuuming plus disposal of bag.
  - ○ Insecticides applied to the environment as powders or sprays:
    Desiccating agents – sodium borate.
    Insect growth regulators – methoprene, fenoxycarb, cyromazine.
    Adulticides – dichlorvos, permethrin.
  - ○ Systemic treatment given to cat as liquid or injection:
    Insect growth regulators – lufenuron (Program, Novartis).
- Control of fleas on the animal.
  - ○ Sprays:
    Dichlorvos/fenitrothion (Nuvan Top, Novartis).
    Fipronil (Frontline, Merial).
  - ○ Spot-on:
    Fipronil (Frontline, Merial).
    Imidocloprid (Advantage, Bayer).
  - ○ Collars, shampoos, powders – limited use.

Anti-inflammatories

- Glucocorticoids.
  - ○ Prednisolone – 1–2 mg/kg daily for 7–10 days, then tapering to lowest possible alternate day dosage.
    Short courses only should be required if flea control is rigorous.
- Antihistamines – limited usage.

Hyposensitisation – success questionable

LICE

Pediculosis

- Uncommon pruritic skin disease caused by lice.

Cause and pathogenesis

- Two suborders:
  - ○ Mallophaga – biting lice – *Felicola subrostratus*.
  - ○ Anoplura – sucking lice – no feline biting lice found in the UK.
- Disease seen especially in winter – lice killed by high skin temperatures.
- Biting lice move rapidly and can be difficult to find and capture.

- Predisposing factors:
  - ○ Young animals – poor hygiene, nutrition, overcrowding.
  - ○ Old animals – systemic disease.

Clinical signs

- Location – especially body openings, ear tips, matted areas of hair on body.
- Pruritus variable – can be asymptomatic carriers, can present as seborrhoea.
- Papular eruptions in sensitive animals leading to self-excoriation.
- Often presents as miliary dermatitis or other component of eosinophilic allergic syndrome (Fig. 5.25).

Differential diagnosis

- Flea allergic dermatitis.
- Cheyletiellosis.
- Allergy – especially atopy, food.
- Trombiculiasis.

Distinguishing features (Figs 5.26–5.28)

- Small dorsoventrally flattened wingless insects 2–3 mm in length.
- Six legs, broad head, three segmented antennae at side of head.

Life cycle – host specific

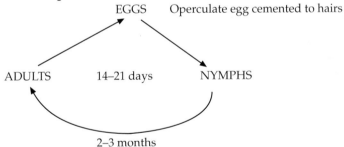

EGGS   Operculate egg cemented to hairs

ADULTS   14–21 days   NYMPHS

2–3 months

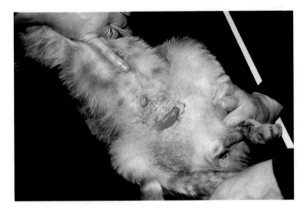

Fig. 5.25 Eosinophilic granuloma secondary to lice infestation.

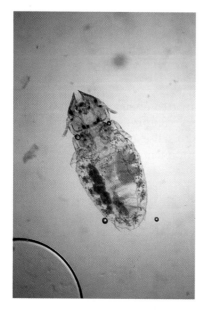

Fig. 5.26 *Felicola subrostratus* – biting louse.

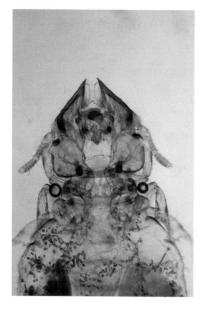

Fig. 5.27 Close up of head of *Felicola*.

Diagnosis

- Clinical signs.
- Identification – acetate tapes to immobilise the lice or superficial skin scrapings.
- Samples should be taken from predilection sites, e.g. ear tips.
- Histopathology unspecific and non-diagnostic.

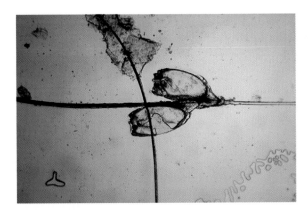

Fig. 5.28 Lice eggs cemented to hair shafts.

Treatment

- Identification and treatment of any underlying factors.
- Clip coat to remove thick crusts and mats to allow penetration and treatment.
- Coat should be soaked or sprayed with a good insecticide.
- No products are specifically licensed for the treatment of lice in cats.
  - ○ Insecticidal shampoo.
    Selenium sulphide 1% (Seleen, Sanofi) – three treatments at 10 day intervals.
  - ○ Sprays:
    Dichlorvos/fenitrothion (Nuvan top, Novartis).
    Fipronil (Frontline, Merial).
- Environmental treatment including grooming equipment, using products suitable for environmental flea control.

FLIES

Mosquito dermatitis

Cause and pathogenesis

- Lesions are seen in cats that are hypersensitive to mosquito bites.
- Lesions resolve without treatment when cats are confined to a mosquito-free environment.

Clinical signs

- Lesions are seen in cats spending time outdoors.
- Seasonality is related to mosquito feeding times.
- Commonly affects bridge of nose, medial aspect of ear pinnae; also footpads, lips and chin.
- Acute lesions range from erythematous plaques and papules to ulcerated erosions.

- Chronic lesions – scaling, alopecia and nodules, often with pigment changes.
- Systemic signs include lymphadenopathy and pyrexia.

Differential diagnosis

- Pemphigus foliaceus/erythematosus.
- Allergy (atopy, food, flea).
- Dermatophytosis.
- Demodicosis.

Diagnosis

- Clinical signs with history of exposure to mosquito bites.
- Resolution of lesions occurs when cat is hospitalised or with the use of repellents.
- Histopathology reveals non-specific changes of eosinophilic infiltrates with collagen degeneration.

Treatment

- Prevention of mosquito bites by:
  - ○ Hospitalisation/confinement during high risk periods.
  - ○ Insect repellents applied to short and sparsely haired areas.
- Treatment of the bites.
  - ○ 7–10 days of anti-inflammatory doses of prednisolone – 1–2 mg/kg once daily.
  - ○ Courses can be extended and used on an alternate day basis for cats who have continual re-exposure.
  - ○ As a seasonal problem steroid therapy should only needed for short periods.

Fly dermatitis

Cause and pathogenesis

- Uncommon pruritic skin disease caused by biting flies, usually on outdoors or farm cats.
- Important flies include:
  - ○ *Stomoxys calcitrans* (stable fly).
  - ○ *Simulium* spp. (black fly).
  - ○ *Tabanus* spp. (horse fly).
  - ○ *Chrysops* spp. (deer fly).

Clinical signs

- Bites usually occur on the face, ears (*Stomoxys calcitrans*), ventral abdomen, legs, and ears (*Simulium* spp.).
- Haemorrhagic papules and crusts.
- Pruritus variable.

Differential diagnosis

- Other ectoparasitic diseases.

Diagnosis

- History, especially exposure to flies.
- Elimination of other causes.

Treatment

- Fly avoidance – source of flies should be identified (knowledge of fly life cycle important).
- Change of housing.
- Fly repellents.
- Treatment of lesions – topical antibiotics and/or corticosteroid preparations.

Myiasis (fly strike)

Cause and pathogenesis

- Infestation of skin with maggots from dipterous flies.
- Flies attracted to warm wet skin, especially urine/faecal stained areas, as well as draining wounds.
- Flies involved
  - Primary flies – initiate strike, especially *Lucilia* spp. and *Calliphora* spp.
  - Secondary flies – larvae extend lesions: *Chrysomyia* spp., *Sarcophaga*.
  - Tertiary flies – last to invade, cause further inflammation, e.g. *Musca* spp.

Predisposing factors

- Poor hygiene.
- Debilitation due to age or illness.
- Urine/faecal incontinence.

Clinical signs

- Lesions affect skin around nose, eyes, mouth, anus and genitalia.
- Punched out holes with tissue necrosis containing larvae (Fig. 5.29).

Diagnosis

- Identification of larvae in wounds.

Treatment

- Treatment of predisposing factors important.
- Clip hair from lesions.
- Clean area with antibacterial wash, e.g. chlorhexidine.
- Surgical debridement may be necessary.

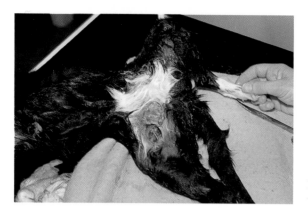

Fig. 5.29 Fly strike involving ventral abdominal skin.

- Remove all larvae.
- Insecticidal wash on area and rest of coat, e.g. selenium sulphide.
- Antibiotics based on culture and sensitivity if necessary.

Cuterebriasis

Cause and pathogenesis

- Infection of skin with larvae of *Cuterebria* spp.
- Cats in warm climates affected (cats imported into the UK).
- Cats are contaminated by picking up eggs laid by adult flies in environment – close to burrows or nests of rabbits or rodents.
- Larvae penetrate the skin or are ingested during grooming.
- Aberrant migration occurs in unnatural host.

Clinical signs

- Lesions found around the head, neck and trunk.
- Nodular swelling approximately 1 cm across with a central air hole and fistula.
- Distant lesions can occur in brain, pharynx, nostrils and eyelids.

Differential diagnosis

- Neoplasia.
- Myiasis.

Diagnosis

- History of exposure.
- Identification of larvae in lesions.

Treatment

- Incision of air hole and gentle extraction of larvae.
- Risk of anaphylaxis if larvae are crushed or incompletely removed.

HYMENOPTERA (BEES, WASPS, HORNETS)

Stings

- Local inflammatory reaction caused by these venomous non-parasitic insects.

Cause and pathogenesis

- Toxin released into the skin as insect stings, leading to local or systemic signs.
- Severity depends on number of stings and animal sensitivity.

Clinical signs

- Mild cases – localised redness, oedema.
- Severe cases – angioedema, anaphylaxis leading to death can occur.

Differential diagnosis

- Other causes of urticaria.

Diagnosis

- Clinical signs and history of exposure to venomous insect.

Treatment

- Localised problem – remove sting if possible.
- Short acting glucocorticoid injections followed by antihistamines, e.g. chlorpheniramine (Piriton) – 4–8 mg three times daily.
- Topical antihistamine cream.
- Anaphylaxis should be treated with intramuscular adrenaline and intravenous glucocorticoids.

HELMINTH PARASITES

NEMATODES

HOOKWORMS

Uncinariasis (hookworm dermatitis)

Cause

- Cutaneous lesions caused by larvae of the hookworm *Uncinaria stenocephala*.
- Rare disease in the cat, seen in Ireland, England and USA.

Table 5.1 Antiparasitic therapy

	Administration/Application	Principal indications
Ectoparasiticides		
Amitraz 5% wash (unlicensed product for cats)	Applied 1:400 diluted with water to whole body weekly	*Demodex*
	Applied 1:400 diluted with water as above	*Notoedres/Sarcoptes*
Dichlorvos/ Fenitrothion spray	Spray time depends on animal size. Every 7–10 days	Fleas
Fipronil - Spray	Applied to whole body (volume depends on pump and animal size)	Fleas, *Cheyletiella*, ticks, *Sarcoptes*, *T. autumnalis*, lice
Spot on	Apply to back of neck dependent on size of cat	Fleas, ticks
Imidocloprid spot on	Apply to back of neck/tail dependent on size of cat	Fleas
Ivermectin injection (unlicensed product for cats)	0.4 mg/kg daily orally (test dose see text) until 30 days beyond clinical cure (up to 200 days)	*Demodex*
	0.3 mg/kg subcutaneously every 7 days for 4 applications	*Notoedres/Sarcoptes*
Selenium sulphide 1% shampoo (unlicensed product for cats)	Whole body shampoo every 10 days for 3 applications	Lice, *Cheyletiella*
Environmental products		
Lufenuron tablets	Monthly oral administration or 6 monthly injections	Fleas
Permethrin/ cyromazine	Environmental spray	Fleas
Pyrethrin/methoprene	Environmental spray	Fleas

Pathogenesis

- Penetration of the skin by the third stage larva of *Uncinaria stenocephala* leads to cutaneous lesions at contact sites.
- Hookworm rarely completes its life cycle by this route.
- Larvae found in soil spring and autumn – cool climates.
- Outdoor and/or cattery animals on grass, soil runs.

Clinical signs

- Papular eruptions on contact sites with ground.
- Chronic lesions – erythema, swelling, alopecia plus digital hyperkeratosis.
- Pruritus variable.

Differential diagnosis

- Contact dermatitis.
- Other causes of foot pad hyperkeratosis.

Diagnosis

- History, poor housing, sanitation.
- Clinical signs.
- Faecal examination for hookworm eggs.

Treatment

- Improvement of hygiene; faeces removal in runs.
- Dry paved runs, or gravel treated with 4.5 kg borax per 30 m^2.
- Anthelmintics – fenbendazole (Panacur, Hoechst) can be used for treatment and prophylaxis.

Ancylostomiasis

- Dermatitis caused by larvae of *Ancylostoma braziliense, A. caninum*.
- Found in warm climates.
- Causes cutaneous lesions less commonly than *Uncinaria stenocephala*.
- Clinical signs, diagnosis and treatment as for *Uncinaria stenocephela*.

Chapter 6

Viral, Rickettsial and Protozoal Diseases

VIRAL DISEASES

- Leukaemia virus.
- Giant cell dermatosis.
- Immunodeficiency virus.
- Pox virus.
- Infectious peritonitis.
- Pseudorabies.
- Rhinotracheitis.
- Calicivirus.
- Papillomavirus.
- Sarcoma virus.

Feline leukaemia virus (FeLV)

Cause and pathogenesis

- Feline leukaemia virus is an oncogenic retrovirus that causes immunosuppression leading to the formation of skin tumours and chronic infection.

Clinical signs

- Skin tumours – lymphoma, fibrosarcoma (see Chapter 18)
- Cutaneous horn – firm horn-like projections usually seen on footpads, occasionally on face. Often cutaneous marker for FeLV.
- Immunosuppression can lead to:
  - Bacterial infection – gingivitis, folliculitis, paronychia (Fig. 6.1), abscesses (Fig. 6.2) especially in cases of atypical mycobacterium, nocardia. May present as non-healing wounds.
  - Yeast/fungal infection – dermatophytosis, *Malassezia*, cryptococcus. Infection often poorly responsive or relapsing.
  - Viral infection – especially cow pox (Fig. 6.3)
  - Parasites – especially demodicosis.

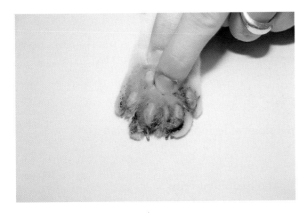

Fig. 6.1 Bacterial paronychia in cat with FeLV.

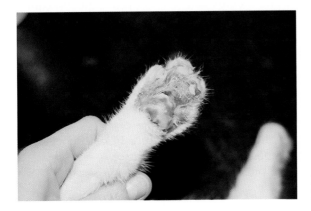

Fig. 6.2 Abscess on paw in FeLV positive cat.

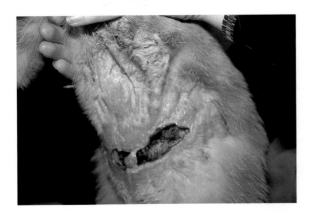

Fig. 6.3 Extensive lesions of cat pox in an FeLV positive cat.

Differential diagnosis

- Any bacterial, fungal, viral or ectoparasitic disease which is poorly responsive to appropriate therapy or where unusual organisms are isolated.

Diagnosis

- Serological tests for FeLV.
- Specific investigations of dermatological lesions as appropriate.

Treatment

- Usually palliative and symptomatic treatment only.
- The response to therapy should where possible be based on appropriate culture and sensitivity.
- Bactericidal and fungicidal therapy offer the best chance of success.
- Some cases respond completely and therapy can be withdrawn; others require long-term treatment.
- Immunosuppressive therapy in the form of glucocorticoids should be avoided.

Giant cell dermatosis

Cause and pathogenesis

- Infection with FeLV is thought to cause neoplastic alteration of keratinocytes by recombination with host's oncogenes, leading to skin disease.

Clinical signs

- No breed or sex predilection.
- All reported cases have been less than 6 years of age.
- Crusting and scaling with diffuse alopecia.
- Variable distribution – ears and periauricular skin commonly involved (Figs 6.4, 6.5).

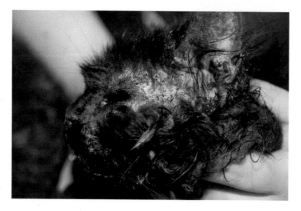

Fig. 6.4 Lesions of giant cell dermatosis affecting the face.

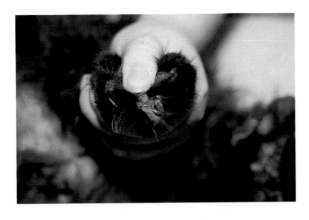

Fig. 6.5 Lesions of giant cell dermatosis affecting the nail beds.

Differential diagnosis

- Dermatophytosis.
- Neoplasia – lymphoma, thymoma.
- Primary seborrhoea.
- *Cheyletiella*.

Diagnosis

- Rule outs including fungal culture and skin scrapings.
- Biopsy – typical syncytial type giant cells.
- Positive immunohistochemistry for FeLV antigen in epidermis and follicles.

Treatment

- No response to antibacterial or antifungal therapy.
- Poor prognosis – most cats euthanased.

Feline immunodeficiency virus (FIV)

Cause and pathogenesis

- A retrovirus capable of producing cytosuppression.
- Clinical signs overlap with those of FeLV infections.

Clinical signs

- See FeLV and Fig. 6.6.
- The clinical signs associated with FIV infection are clinically similar to those of FeLV and can only be differentiated by serological identification of the virus involved.
- The two viruses can occur concurrently leading to synergistic immunosuppression.

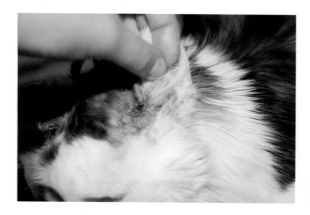

Fig. 6.6 Pyoderma in an FIV positive cat.

Differential diagnosis

- As FeLV.

Diagnosis

- Serological tests for FIV.

Treatment

- As FeLV.

Feline pox virus

Cause and pathogenesis

- Feline pox virus is a member of the *Orthopoxvirus* genus.
- Small wild rodents are thought to be the reservoir for infection – cats become infected through a bite wound.
- Disease is seen in numerous European countries, including the UK.
- No sex, breed or age incidence recognised, although most cases occur in the autumn.
- Zoonotic disease.

Clinical signs

- Initial lesion is an infected bite wound usually on head (Fig. 6.7) or forelimb.
- Viraemia after local replication leads to the formation of multiple secondary lesions.
- Secondary lesions appear as ulcerated papules and nodules leading to crusted sores (Fig. 6.8).
- Appearance of non-allergic miliary dermatitis.
- Pruritus variable but can be intense.
- Systemic signs rare unless cat immunosuppressed.

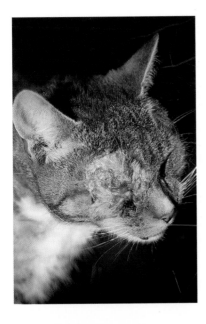

Fig. 6.7 Primary bite wound thought to be from a rodent in a case of cat pox.

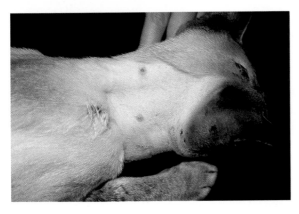

Fig. 6.8 Secondary miliary lesions in cat pox.

Differential diagnosis

- Dermatophytosis.
- Eosinophilic granuloma complex.
- Allergic miliary dermatitis.
- Neoplasia (lymphoma, mast cell tumour).

Diagnosis

- Clinical signs and history.
- Electron microscopy of scabs for virus.
- Virus isolation from tissue or scabs (submitted to an appropriate laboratory in viral transport medium).

- Biopsy – histopathology may reveal characteristic intracytoplasmic inclusions.
- Serology (specialised laboratories only).

Treatment

- Lesions will heal slowly over 3–4 weeks without therapy in an uncomplicated case.
- If secondary infection is present antibiotics should be prescribed based on culture and sensitivity where possible.
- Empirical therapy can be undertaken with cephalexin, clindamycin or clavamox (see Table 2.1 for dose rates).
- Where the cat is pruritic symptomatic therapy can be given with antihistamines:
  - Chlorpheniramine – 4 mg per cat by mouth two or three times daily.
  - Promethazine – 12.5 mg per cat by mouth twice daily.
- An Elizabethan collar can be used to prevent self-traumatisation.
- Glucocorticoids are contraindicated.
- In immunosuppressed or systemically unwell cats supportive therapy is also required.
- Euthanasia is often necessary in severe cases.

Feline infectious peritonitis (FIP)

Cause and pathogenesis

- A multisystemic viral disease caused by a coronavirus.
- Systemic disease can be effusive (exudate found in body cavities) and/or non-effusive (pyogranulomatous lesions in various sites).

Clinical signs

- Systemic disease.
- Usually affects abdominal organs – often abdominal distension, also ocular and neurological signs.
- Cutaneous lesions.
- Usually associated with debilitation and ataxia.
- Ulcerative lesions around the head and neck have been seen in experimentally infected cats.

Diagnosis

- Clinical signs.
- Positive FIP titre in combination with supportive serum chemistry, haematology and fluid analysis.

Treatment

- Symptomatic and supportive therapy.

Pseudorabies ('Mad itch')

Cause and pathogenesis

- Fatal rare severely pruritic skin disease caused by alpha-herpes virus.
- Pigs are reservoirs of infection.
- Cats infected by contact with infected animals or by eating infected raw pork.

Clinical signs

- Systemic signs.
- Rare acute cases – coma and death.
- More commonly – excessive salivation, restlessness, neurological signs including ataxia.
- Cutaneous lesions.
- Intense pruritus of upper body – especially face and mouth.

Differential diagnosis

- Rabies.
- Ectoparasiticism – especially scabies.
- Allergies, e.g. atopy, food allergy.

Diagnosis

- Clinical signs and history of contact with infected animals.
- Isolation of virus from nervous tissue at the site of pruritus.
- Cats normally die before circulating antibodies appear.
- Virus isolation – swabs in transport medium.

Treatment

- No treatment available.
- Source of infection should be identified.

Feline rhinotracheitis

Cause and pathogenesis

- Very common disease caused by a herpes virus (feline herpes virus 1, FHV1).
- Route of infection is intranasal, oral or conjunctival.
- Upper respiratory tract signs most common – especially seen in young and immunosuppressed cats.

Clinical signs

- Systemic signs:
  - Ocular and nasal discharge with conjunctivitis (Fig. 6.9).

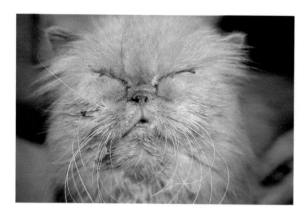

Fig. 6.9 Ocular and nasal discharge in a cat with herpesvirus.

- ○ Oral ulceration leading to hypersalivation.
- ○ Severe cases dyspnoea and coughing.
- Cutaneous signs – uncommon:
  - ○ Superficial ulcers can occur anywhere on the body especially footpads.
  - ○ Periocular alopecia.
  - ○ Ulcers can be precipitated by stress or trauma.

Differential diagnosis

- Systemic signs – other causes of upper respiratory tract disease.
- Cutaneous signs:
  - ○ Vasculitis.
  - ○ Drug eruptions.
  - ○ Erythema multiforme.
  - ○ Neoplasia (lymphoma).

Diagnosis

- Clinical signs in an unvaccinated cat.
- Oropharyngeal or skin swabs in viral transport medium.
- Biopsy.
  - ○ Histopathology may reveal basophilic intranuclear inclusions.
  - ○ Electron microscopy to identify virus in keratinocytes.

Treatment

- Topical antiviral eye preparations for ocular signs.
- Broad spectrum antibiotic therapy for secondary bacterial involvement.
- Symptomatic therapy for systemically unwell cats.
- Glucocorticoids are contraindicated.

Feline calicivirus

Cause and pathogenesis

- Common viral disease caused by a calicivirus.
- Infection occurs by the oral, intranasal or conjunctival routes.
- Upper respiratory and oral cavity signs occur most commonly.

Clinical signs

- Oral lesions very common (Fig. 6.10). These start as vesicles (Fig. 6.11) that rupture to form ulcers.
- Cutaneous ulceration also been reported on feet and perineum.
- Ocular, nasal, conjunctival and pulmonary disease less severe than FHV1.

Differential diagnosis

- Other causes of oral ulceration:
  - ○ Pemphigus vulgaris.
  - ○ Bacterial stomatitis.

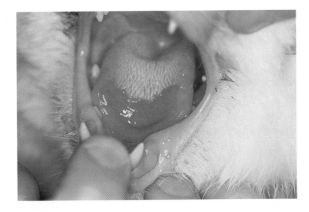

Fig. 6.10 Oral ulceration in a cat with calicivirus infection (picture courtesy of D. Crossley).

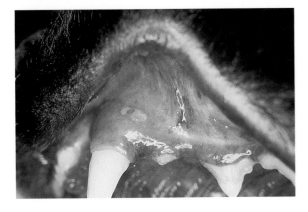

Fig. 6.11 Vesicles on the gums of a cat with calicivirus infection (picture courtesy of D. Crossley).

○ Drug eruption.
○ Systemic lupus erythematosus.

Diagnosis

- Clinical signs in an unvaccinated cat, especially where oral ulceration predominates.
- Oropharyngeal or skin swabs in viral transport medium.

Treatment

- As FHV1.

Papillomavirus

Cause and pathogenesis

- Rare disease caused by papilloma virus.
- Thought to cause flat warts in some cats and may be implicated in 'feline sarcoids'.

Clinical signs

Viral squamous papillomas (flat warts)

- Multiple randomly scattered black circular plaques found on forelegs, head and shoulders.
- Old Persians predisposed.
- May occur secondary to immune dysfunction.

Fibropapilloma (feline sarcoid)

- Well circumscribed proliferative lesions, can occur at any site.
- No age, breed or sex predilection.

Differential diagnosis

Viral squamous papilloma

- Neoplasia – especially squamous cell carcinoma.
- Cutaneous horn.

Fibropapilloma

- Collagenous naevus.
- Neoplasia.
- Granulation tissue.
- Eosinophilic granuloma.

Diagnosis

- Clinical signs.
- Biopsy squamous papilloma.
  - ○ Intracytoplasmic inclusions on histopathology.
  - ○ Papillomavirus virions in nuclei visible by electron microscopy.
  - ○ Immunoperoxidase stains for virus.
- Biopsy fibropapilloma.
  - ○ Virus has not been identified.

Treatment

- Surgical excision usually curative.

Feline sarcoma virus

- Sarcoma virus has been associated with the formation of cutaneous fibrosarcomas in young cats (see Chapter 18).

RICKETTSIAL DISEASES

Haemobartonellosis (feline infectious anaemia)

Cause and pathogenesis

- Acute or chronic disease caused by parasitism of the red blood cells by *Haemobartonella felis*.

Clinical signs

- Systemic signs – those caused by anaemia, i.e. lethargy, weight loss.
- Cutaneous signs – hyperaesthesia and alopecia areata have been reported.

Diagnosis

- Clinical signs.
- Haematology – macrocytic haemolytic anaemia.
- Identification of causal organism on stained blood films.

Treatment

- Supportive therapy for anaemia dependent on severity.
- Antibiotics.
  - ○ Oxytetracycline – 20 mg/kg by mouth three times daily for a minimum of 14 days.

PROTOZOAL DISEASES

- Toxoplasmosis.
- Leishmaniasis.

Toxoplasmosis

Cause and pathogenesis

- Multisystemic disease caused by the protozoan parasite *Toxoplasma gondii.*

Clinical signs

- Systemic signs:
  - Very variable and can affect any organ system.
  - Acute disease – pyrexia, hepatitis, pneumonia.
  - Chronic disease – anaemia, iritis, encephalitis.
- Cutaneous signs:
  - Nodular lesions on the legs.

Diagnosis

- Clinical signs.
- Skin biopsy.
  - Necrotising dermatitis and vasculits.
  - Organisms seen in stained tissue sections.

Treatment

- Trimethoprim/sulphonamide.
  - Dosage as mg of total product.
  - 15 mg/kg by mouth twice daily/for 10–14 days.

Leishmaniasis

Cause and pathogenesis

- Very rare disease in the cat caused by *Leishmania* spp.
- Seen in Mediterranean countries, Central America, parts of Africa, Middle East and imported cats in UK.
- Zoonotic disease.
- Disease transmitted by blood sucking sand flies, usually *Phlebotomus*.
- Mediterranean areas – *L. donovani* most important.
- Incubation period weeks–years.

Clinical signs

- Systemic signs – weight loss, pyrexia, hepato-splenomegaly, lameness.
- Cutaneous signs – nodules or crusted ulcers on the lips, nose, eyelids and pinnae.

Differential diagnosis

- Pemphigus foliaceus.
- Systemic lupus erythematosus.
- Dermatophytosis.
- Eosinophilic granuloma complex.
- Neoplasia (lymphoma).

Diagnosis

- History and clinical signs – especially in imported cats in UK.
- Serology – anti-Leishmania antibodies.
- Smear from bone marrow or lymph nodes demonstrates amastigotes.
- Skin biopsy organism identified inside macrophages.
- Immunohistochemistry.

Treatment

- Poor prognosis.
- Relapses common – therefore euthanasia should be considered.
- Successful treatment for feline leishmaniasis has not been reported.

Chapter 7

Immunological Skin Diseases

HYPERSENSITIVITY DISORDERS

Urticaria and angioedema

Cause and pathogenesis

- Immunological or non-immunological degranulation of mast cells or basophils.
- Immunological trigger type I, III hypersensitivity reaction.
- Non-immunological:
  - Physical forces (pressure).
  - Genetic abnormalities.
  - Drugs and chemicals.
- Both urticaria and angioedema are rare diseases in the cat.

Clinical signs

Urticaria

- Localised or generalised wheals.
- Pruritus and exudation variable.
- Hair tufts over areas of swelling.
- Generally benign self-limiting disease.

Angioedema

- Localised or generalised area of large oedematous swelling.
- Pruritus and exudation variable.
- May be fatal if oedema involves pharynx and larynx.

Differential diagnosis

- Dermatophytosis.
- Miliary dermatitis.
- Eosinophilic granuloma complex.
- Vasculitis.
- Erythema multiforme.
- Neoplasia (lymphoma, mast cell tumours).

Diagnosis

- History.
- Physical examination.
- Identification of triggers – not always possible.
- Skin biopsy – variable, non-diagnostic pattern.

Treatment

- Elimination and avoidance of trigger factors.
- Treatment of symptoms with:
  - ○ Adrenalin 1:1000 – 0.1–0.5 ml subcutaneously.
  - ○ Glucocorticoids – prednisolone – 2 mg/kg by mouth, intravenously or intramuscularly.
  - ○ Antihistamines – variable effectiveness.
    Chlorpheniramine (Piriton) – 4 mg per cat two or three times daily.

Atopy (Atopic dermatitis)

- An exaggerated or inappropriate response to environmental allergens.

Cause and pathogenesis

- Thought to be an immediate hypersensitivity reaction to a heat labile antibody resembling IgE.
- Route of allergen – percutaneous, inhaled or ingested.

Clinical signs

- No breed or sex predilection.
- Young cats appear to be predisposed.
- Cats are always pruritic.
- Different cutaneous patterns can be seen.
  - ○ Self-induced alopecia (usually ventral and extremities) (Figs 7.1, 7.2).
  - ○ Eosinophilic granuloma complex.
  - ○ Allergic miliary dermatitis.
  - ○ Facial and pedal pruritus (often secondary bacterial paronychia; Fig. 7.3).
  - ○ Pruritic ceruminous otitis externa.
- Many cats have concurrent food hypersensitivity and flea allergic dermatitis.

Differential diagnosis

- Flea allergic dermatitis.
- Food hypersensitivity.
- *Cheyletiella.*
- Ectopic *Otodectes.*
- Dermatophytosis.
- Psychogenic alopecia.

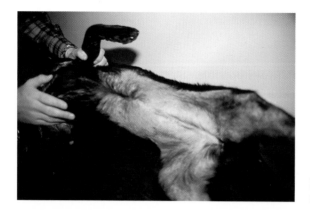

Fig. 7.1 Ventral alopecia secondary to atopy.

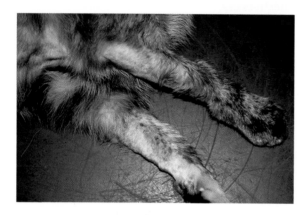

Fig. 7.2 Pedal alopecia secondary to atopy.

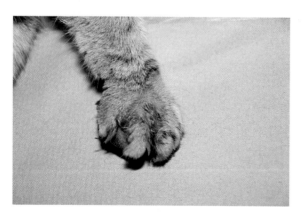

Fig. 7.3 Bacterial paronychia secondary to atopy.

Diagnosis

- History and clinical signs.
- Laboratory rule-outs for other diseases, especially flea/food allergy.
- Intradermal skin testing useful as an aid to diagnosis (Fig. 7.4).

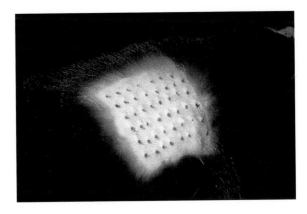

Fig. 7.4 Intradermal skin test in an atopic cat.

- ○ Difficult to undertake in the cat as reactions are more subtle than in the dog.
- ○ Reactions often occur and fade rapidly within 10 minutes.
- ○ Must be read by an experienced investigator.
- Serology testing not adequately evaluated to date.
- Skin biopsy – usually non-specific, acts as a rule-out rather than as a diagnosis.
- Bloods – peripheral eosinophilia usually present unless glucocorticoids have been prescribed.

Treatment

- Treatment usually required for life.
- Avoidance – often not possible but exposure can decrease significantly through environmental changes.
- Topical therapy – rarely undertaken due to difficulty in bathing cats.
  - ○ Where cat and owner are willing it can be useful.
  - ○ Antipruritic agents include colloidal oatmeal (Episoothe, Virbac; Dermasooth, C Vet).
- Hyposensitisation.
  - ○ Useful in cats where allergen avoidance is impossible and where topical and systemic treatment is unsatisfactory.
  - ○ Success rate 50–80%.
  - ○ Effective, valuable and relatively safe treatment for atopic cats.
  - ○ Should be considered as an option to injectable steroids in cats that are difficult to medicate.
- Systemic antipruritic drugs.
  - ○ Antihistamines have been shown to be useful.
    Clemastine (Tavegil) – 0.67 mg per cat orally twice daily.
    Chlorpheniramine (Piriton) – 2.0 mg per cat twice daily.
    Response to various drugs is individual and unpredictable.
  - ○ Essential fatty acid supplementation.
    Products containing both omega-3 and omega-6 fatty acids have been shown to be useful.
    Additive effects noted with both glucocorticoids and antihistamines.

○ Systemic glucocorticoids.
  Prednisolone – 1 mg/kg once daily until signs controlled in 7–10 days, then on alternate days at the lowest possible dose for maintenance.
  Methylprednisolone acetate – 5 mg/kg intramuscularly can be used in cats who are difficult with tablets. It should not be given more than four times a year and should never replace a more thorough investigation.

Contact hypersensitivity

- Very rare dermatitis manifested usually as an allergic maculopapular reaction affecting sparsely haired contact areas.

Cause and pathogenesis

- Contact allergy – type IV hypersensitivity reaction, must be distinguished from contact irritants.
- Triggered by plants, metals, rubber, resins, and carpet deodorisers.
- Topical hypersensitivity reactions to drugs also occur – neomycin.

Clinical signs

- No breed predilection.
- Single animal in household affected suggests hypersensitivity – several animals affected suggests irritancy.
- Sensitisation period usually 2 years or more.
- Lesions confined to hairless/sparsely haired areas, except where signs caused by creams, shampoos, etc., especially ventral abdomen, thorax, neck, perineum, ventral aspect of paws (not pads).
- Acute – erythema, papules, pustules variable.
- Chronic – alopecia (Fig. 7.5), variable pigment changes (hypo- or hyperpigmentation), lichenification.

Differential diagnosis

- Irritant contact dermatitis.
- Atopy.
- Food hypersensitivity.
- Flea allergic dermatitis.

Diagnosis

- History and clinical signs.
- Provocative exposure.
  ○ Animal confined to hypoallergenic environment for 14 days.
  ○ Careful re-exposure to potential allergens to try and trigger reaction.
- Patch testing.
  ○ Closed patch test.

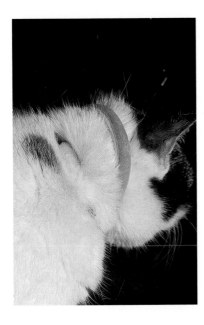

Fig. 7.5 Chronic contact hypersensitivity due to a flea collar.

> Test substance applied to clipped skin on lateral thorax on gauze pad or in Finn chamber, secured in place by a body bandage.
> Examination after 48 hours reveals signs of hypersensitive reaction.
> ○ Open patched test.
> Test substance rubbed into skin and then observed over a 5 day period.
- Skin biopsy – non diagnostic.

Treatment

- Allergen avoidance.
- Glucocorticoids often needed long term.
- Systemic treatment – prednisolone – 1 mg/kg by mouth on alternate days.
- Topical treatment – use of potent steroids should be avoided because of cutaneous absorption.

Food hypersensitivity (Food intolerance/food allergy)

- Non-seasonal pruritic skin disease associated with ingestion of components of the diet.

Cause and pathogenesis

- Pathogenesis poorly understood.
- Food allergy occurs – especially type I reactions to food.
- Food intolerance clinically indistinguishable from allergy, but non-immunological reaction. Caused by food containing histamine or related substances; histamine releasing factors also important.

- Foods implicated in hypersensitivity include dairy products, fish, beef, pork, chicken, lamb and eggs.

Clinical signs

- No age or sex predilection – often seen in cats 4–5 years of age.
- Siamese cats may be predisposed.
- Pruritus seen in 100% of cases, and is non-seasonal.
- Cutaneous signs variable.
- Different reaction patterns are recognised.
  - Most common signs are:
    Facial pruritus, including pinnae and neck (Fig. 7.6).
    Ventral or flank alopecia (self-inflicted due to over grooming).
    Allergic miliary dermatitis.
    Eosinophilic granuloma complex (Fig. 7.7).
  - Less common signs include:
    Papulopustular eruptions.
    Urticaria.

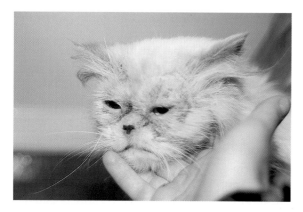

Fig. 7.6 Facial pruritus secondary to food allergy.

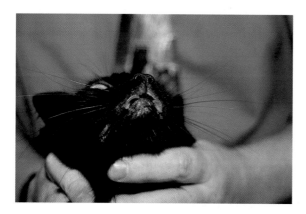

Fig. 7.7 Indolent ulcer in a food allergic cat.

○ Non-cutaneous signs are:
Gastrointestinal signs – diarrhoea and vomiting.
Sneezing, dullness.
- 25% of cases have other concurrent allergies.

Differential diagnosis

- Depends on the clinical signs but should include:
  ○ Atopy.
  ○ Flea allergic dermatitis.
  ○ Psychogenic alopecia.
  ○ Dermatophytosis.
  ○ Ectopic *Otodectes*.
  ○ Cheyletiellosis.
  ○ Pediculosis.

Diagnosis

- History and clinical signs.
- Response to elimination diet which should be fed for a minimum of 4 weeks and up to 12 weeks in some cases.
- Some improvement should be seen in 4 weeks.
- Selection of diet.
  ○ Individualised for each cat – dependent on previous dietary history.
  ○ Novel protein sources include duck, turkey, soya, venison.
  ○ Free of additives, colourants, etc., if possible.
- Types of diet.
  ○ Home cooked ideal – owner compliance often poor, unbalanced for cats for long term usage. Supplementation with, e.g. taurine or calcium, may be necessary.
  ○ Commercial hypoallergenic diets – not a 'pure' diet but more convenient for busy owners and are nutritionally complete.
- Cat should be kept inside during food trial.
- Laboratory tests.
  ○ Scratch, intradermal and serological tests are unreliable.
- Skin biopsy – not diagnostic.

Treatment

- Allergen avoidance.
  ○ Reintroduction of different foods to hypoallergenic diet allows offending allergens to be identified.
  ○ Each new challenge food should be added every 7–10 days.
- Selection of diet long term.
  ○ Home cooked with additional minerals, vitamins and essential fatty acid supplements.
  ○ Proprietary diets that do not contain any of the identified allergens.
- Glucocorticoids, antihistamines of limited benefit.

Parasitic hypersensitivity

- Flea allergic dermatitis – see Chapter 5.
- Other ectoparasitic hypersensitivities.
- Cutaneous hypersensitivity appears to be important in other ectoparasitic infestations.
  - ○ Tick bite hypersensitivity.
  - ○ Otodectic mange.

AUTOIMMUNE SKIN DISEASE

Pemphigus complex

- Very rare vesiculobullous pustular diseases of the skin and mucous membranes.
- Many different forms are recognised.
  - ○ Pemphigus vulgaris.*
  - ○ Pemphigus vegetans.
  - ○ Pemphigus foliaceus.*
  - ○ Pemphigus erythematosus.*
  - ○ IgA pemphigus.
  - ○ Paraneoplastic pemphigus.
- Pemphigus can be associated with drugs (including food substances), chronic disease and immune system related tumours.

Pemphigus vulgaris

Cause and pathogenesis

- Autoantibodies react with 130 kD glycoprotein from the cadherin group of adhesion molecules.[†]
- Results in loss of intercellular cohesion and acantholysis at the suprabasilar level.

Clinical signs

- Second rarest form of pemphigus.
- No age, breed or sex predilection.
- Cutaneous signs.
  - ○ Vesicles, bullae, erosions, ulcers found in oral cavity (90%) and mucocutaneous junctions.

---

*Described in the cat.
†Pathomechanism as described in man.

○ Occasionally lesions seen in groin and axilla.
○ Ulcerative paronychia and onychomadesis.
○ Nikolsky sign may be present.
- Non-cutaneous signs.
  ○ Anorexia, pyrexia.

Differential diagnosis

- Systemic lupus erythematosus.
- Cat flu, especially calicivirus infection.
- Toxic epidermal necrolysis.
- Drug eruption.
- Erythema multiforme.
- Bacterial stomatitis.

Diagnosis

- Clinical signs.
- Skin biopsy of primary lesion where possible – suprabasilar acantholysis 'tombstones' of basement membrane.

Treatment

- Very poor prognosis – without treatment this disease is fatal.
- Difficult to achieve and maintain cats in remission.
- Cats are susceptible to azathioprine toxicity (severe bone marrow suppression); therefore chlorambucil is used in combination with prednisolone.
- Combination immunosuppressive therapy usually required.
  ○ Prednisolone – 4.0–8.0 mg/kg by mouth once daily.
  ○ Chlorambucil – 0.1–0.2 mg/kg every 24–48 hours.
  ○ Both drugs are given together to achieve clinical remission and then tapered to lowest possible alternate day dosage of each.
- Long term monitoring.
- Prednisolone therapy – urine for glucosuria, haematuria.
- Chlorambucil – every 2 weeks complete blood count and platelet count until maintenance; then two or three times yearly.

Pemphigus vegetans

Cause and pathogenesis

- A more benign form of pemphigus vulgaris in animals that show less autoreactivity.

Clinical signs

- Not recorded in the cat.
- Cutaneous signs in the dog – verrucous vegetations and papillomatous proliferations.

Differential diagnosis

- Bacterial granulomas.
- Fungal granulomas.
- Cutaneous neoplasia – especially epitheliotrophic lymphoma.

Diagnosis

- Skin biopsy – papillomatosis, sterile microabscesses containing eosinophils and acanthocytes.

Treatment

- As pemphigus vulgaris.

Pemphigus foliaceus

Cause and pathogenesis

- Autoantibodies react with 150 kD glycoprotein (desmoglein I) from cadherin group of adhesion molecules.*
- Results in loss of intercellular cohesion and acantholysis at the intragranular or subcorneal level.

Clinical signs

- The most common form of pemphigus complex disease in the cat.
- No age or sex predilection.
- Cutaneous signs:
   ○ Initial signs usually on face – often follow a waxing and waning course.
   ○ Sterile paronychia, with a thick caseous discharge (Fig. 7.8).

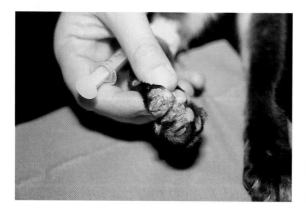

Fig. 7.8 Sterile caseous paronychia in pemphigus foliaceus.

---

*Pathomechanism as described in man.

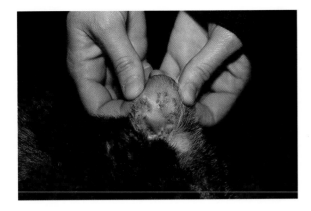

Fig. 7.9 Sterile pustular lesions with pemphigus foliaceus.

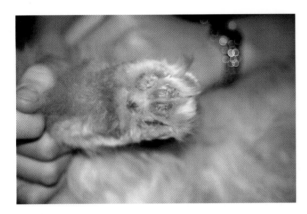

Fig. 7.10 Hyperkeratosis of footpads in pemphigus foliaceus.

- ○ Primary lesions macules and pustules (Fig. 7.9) progressing to severe crusting – non-allergic miliary-dermatitis-like lesions.
  - ○ Involvement of nipples and footpads (Fig. 7.10) common.
  - ○ Nose often depigmented chronically.
  - ○ Claw and oral signs rare.
  - ○ Nikolsky sign may be present.
- Non-cutaneous signs.
  - ○ Anorexic, depression, pyrexia.

Differential diagnosis

- Bacterial impetigo-folliculitis.
- Dermatophytosis.
- Demodicosis.
- Lupus erythematosus.
- Allergy (food, atopy).

Diagnosis

- History and clinical signs.
- Smear of pustules – acanthocytes, non-degenerate neutrophils and/or eosinophils, no bacteria.
- Skin biopsy – intragranular/subcorneal acantholysis with cleft and pustule formation (granular cells 'cling ons').

Treatment

Localised cases

- Topical steroids – risk of iatrogenic Cushing's with long term topical potent steroids.

Generalised disease

- Oral glucocorticoids are drugs of choice.
  Prednisolone – 2.0–6.0 mg/kg by mouth daily tapering to lowest possible alternate day dosage once remission is achieved.
  Dexamethasone – 0.2–0.4 mg/kg by mouth daily tapered to lowest possible dosage every second or third day.
  Triamcinolone – 0.4–0.8 mg/kg by mouth daily tapering (as above).
- 50% of cases require additional immunosuppressive therapy with either chlorambucil or gold.
- Chlorambucil therapy as pemphigus vulgaris.
- Chrysotherapy.
  Gold injection (Solganol, Schering).
  Initially as an intramuscular test dose of 1 mg.
  Then at a dose of 1 mg/kg weekly until remission obtained.
  Lag period for gold is 6–12 weeks; other drugs (e.g. steroids) may have to be maintained during this time.
  After remission the gold is given every 2 weeks.
  Monitoring.
  Induction period – full blood count and urine analysis weekly.
  Long term – monthly blood and urine checks.

Pemphigus erythematosus

Cause and pathogenesis

- Benign form of pemphigus foliaceus – possible cross over between pemphigus and lupus erythematosus.
- Sunlight may play a part in pathogenesis.

Clinical signs

- No age or sex predilection.
- Affects face and ears – pustules, leading to crusts, scale and erosion.
- Nikolsky signs may be present.

- Nose often depigmented chronically.
- No oral signs.

Differential diagnosis

- As pemphigus foliaceus.

Diagnosis

- As pemphigus foliaceus.
- Skin biopsy as pemphigus foliaceus except lichenoid infiltrate often seen at dermoepidermal junction.

Treatment

- Topical steroids.
  - Potent steroid gel/creams initially, e.g. those containing betamethasone (Fuciderm, Leo Labs, Vetsovate, Schering-Plough) until clinical remission is achieved, then less potent steroids used for maintenance, e.g. 1–2% hydrocortisone.
- Systemic steroids.
  - Prednisolone as for pemphigus foliaceus.

IgA pemphigus

- Autoantibodies of IgA group thought to react to desmosomal proteins – desmocollin I and II.*
- Results in intraepidermal pustule formation and acantholysis.
- Presents as a vesiculopustular disease.

Paraneoplastic pemphigus

- Autoantibodies of IgG group react with a complex of four epidermal proteins including desmosomal proteins – desmoplakin I and II.*
- Results in acantholysis together with necrosis and vacuolation of basal layer keratinocytes.
- Lesions can mimic erythema multiforme, pemphigus vulgaris and bullous pemphigoid.
- Associated neoplasms include malignant lymphoma, leukaemia, thymoma and sarcoma.

Systemic lupus erythematosus (SLE)

- Very rare multisystemic autoimmune disease in the cat.

---

*Pathomechanism as described in man.

Cause and pathogenesis

- Multifactorial – genetic susceptibility, immunological factors, drug induction, viral, hormonal and ultraviolet light components are all thought to be important.
- Over-reactive B cells produce antibodies against a variety of body tissues – type III hypersensitivity.
- Skin lesions thought to be caused by autoantibodies to antigens on epidermal basal cells inducing antibody dependent cytotoxicity.

Clinical signs

- No age or sex predilection.
- Predisposed breeds – Siamese, Persian, Himalayan cats.
- Cutaneous lesions seen in about 20% of cases include:
  - Seborrhoeic skin disease.
  - Exfoliative erythroderma.
  - Paronychia.
  - Erythematous, scaling and crusting alopecia involving the head and ears.
- Systemic signs include:
  - Weight loss.
  - Glomerulonephritis.
  - Haemolytic anaemia.
  - Pyrexia.
  - Polyarthritis.
  - Neurological abnormalities.
  - Myopathy.
  - Oral ulceration (Fig. 7.11).

Differential diagnosis

- Almost any skin disease including:
  - Dermatophytosis.
  - Demodicosis.

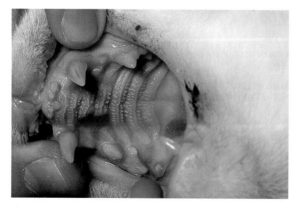

Fig. 7.11 Oral ulceration in a cat with systemic lupus erythematosus (picture courtesy of J. Henfrey).

○ Hypersensitivities (food, fleas, atopy).
○ Pemphigus complex.
○ Epitheliotropic lymphoma.

Diagnosis

- Major and minor diagnostic criteria have not been defined in the cat.
- Recognition of multisystemic disease – especially affecting skin, haematopoietic system, kidney, joints and oral mucosa.
- Serology.
  ○ Positive antinuclear antibody test (ANA).
  ○ False positives can occur, especially in cases of feline infectious peritonitis.
- Cutaneous lupus erythematosus diagnosed by:
  ○ Clinical signs.
  ○ Skin biopsy can be non-diagnostic – however interface dermatitis highly suggestive.

Treatment

- Success of treatment depends on extent of systemic involvement.
- Where haematological abnormalities identified prognosis more guarded.
- Drug therapy.
  ○ Combination therapy with prednisolone and chlorambucil (doses as pemphigus vulgaris).
  ○ Less responsive cases may need dexamethasone or triamcinolone (doses as pemphigus foliaceus) in combination with chlorambucil.
  ○ Methylprednisolone acetate – limited efficacy in SLE.
  ○ Use of megoestrol acetate. In the author's opinion the side effects of this drug in the treatment of this disease outweigh the benefits.

Discoid lupus erythematosus

- Very rare cutaneous autoimmune disease with no systemic involvement.

Cause and pathogenesis

- Type III hypersensitivity reaction caused by autoantibodies to antigens on epithelial basal cells.
- Thought to be aggravated by ultraviolet light.

Clinical signs

- Very few reported cases.
- No age or sex predilection.
- Siamese may be predisposed.
- Lesions generally affect the face (Fig. 7.12).

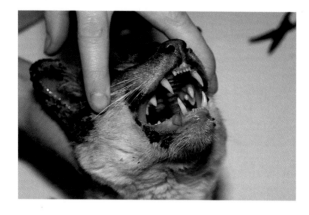

Fig. 7.12 Facial lesions in discoid lupus erythematosus.

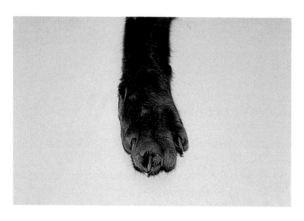

Fig. 7.13 Ulcerative nail bed lesions with discoid lupus erythematosus.

- Erythema, scaling, crusting with ulceration especially pinnae.
- Paronchyia (Fig. 7.13).
- Nasal signs less common.
- Pruritus variable.

Differential diagnosis

- Pemphigus erythematosus/foliaceus.
- Epitheliotrophic lymphoma.
- Drug reaction.
- Dermatophytosis.
- Allergy (food, atopy).

Diagnosis

- History and clinical signs (absence of systemic disease).
- Laboratory tests.
  - ○ ANA usually negative.
  - ○ Blood samples usually unremarkable.

- Skin biopsy – interface dermatitis highly suggestive of discoid lupus erythematosus.

Treatment

- This is not a life threatening disease and carries a good prognosis. Therapy should be prescribed on this basis.
- The use of potent life threatening drugs cannot be justified except in severe recalcitrant cases.
- Sun avoidance from 8.00 a.m. to 5.00 p.m.
- Topical sunscreens and steroids difficult to apply to cats; therefore systemic therapy preferable.
- Systemic steroids.
  - Prednisolone – 2.2–4.4 mg/kg given orally daily. In severe cases this can be given in combination with chlorambucil (see pemphigus vulgaris for dosage).

Cold agglutinin disease

Cause and pathogenesis

- Cryoglobulins and cryofibrinogens precipitate from serum and plasma, respectively, by cooling leading to vascular damage and clinical lesions.
- Type II hypersensitivity associated with cold reacting autoantibodies (usually immunoglobulin M, IgM) to erythrocytes.
- Autoantibodies most active at 0–4°C, although reactions can occur at other temperatures.

Clinical signs

- Underlying causes idiopathic, lead poisoning (usually gunshot wound) or upper respiratory infection.
- Lesions.
  - Acute disease erythema, ulceration of extremities (paws, noses, ear tips, tail) progresses to acrocyanosis (Fig. 7.14).
  - Chronic lesions slough off affected area (Fig. 7.15).
- Signs associated with exposure to cold.

Differential diagnosis

- Vasculitis.
- Systemic lupus erythematosus.
- Frostbite.
- Toxoplasmosis.

Diagnosis

- History and clinical signs – especially exposure to cold.
- Autoagglutination of blood in heparin or EDTA on slide at room temperature.

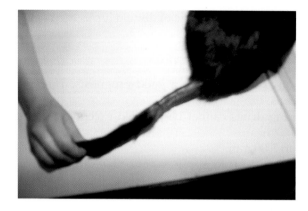

Fig. 7.14 Acrocyanosis of tail tip.

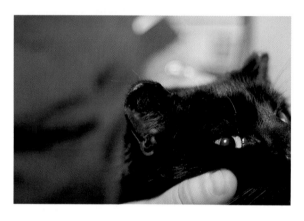

Fig. 7.15 Ear tip slough in cold agglutinin disease.

- Reaction accentuated by cooling to 0°C, reversed on warming to 37°C.
- Positive Coomb's test at 4°C.
- Skin biopsy taken from edge of lesions – thrombosis, vasculitis.

Treatment

- Correction of underlying cause where possible.
- Avoidance of cold.
- Immunosuppression, e.g. glucocorticoids in idiopathic cases probably inappropriate in cases of lead poisoning and respiratory infection.
- The extremity will slough, but once disease controlled will heal uneventfully.

Erythema multiforme

Cause and pathogenesis

- Immunological reaction which can be triggered by:
  ○ Infections.

○ Drugs.*
○ Neoplasia.
○ Connective tissue disorders.
○ Idiopathic.

Clinical signs

- Cutaneous lesions.
  ○ Usually affect mucocutaneous junctions' pinnae, axilla and groin – acute onset.
  ○ Lesions can be variable including erythematous annular 'bulls eyes', urticarial plaques and vesicles and bullae (Fig. 7.16).
- Non-cutaneous lesions.
  ○ Depression, anorexia, pyrexia.

Differential diagnosis

- Dermatophytosis.
- Eosinophilic granuloma complex.
- Miliary dermatitis.
- Urticaria.
- Demodicosis.
- Other vesicular and pustular diseases.

Diagnosis

- History and clinical signs – typical acute onset disease after administration of drug therapy (cephalexin, penicillin and gold reported as inciting drugs).
- Laboratory rule-out of other conditions.
- Skin biopsy – variable picture depending on type of lesion.

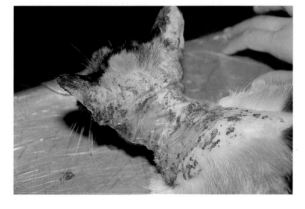

Fig. 7.16 Erythema multiforme caused by carbimazole in a hyperthyroid cat.

---

*Reported in the cat.

Treatment

- Identification of treatment of underlying cause where possible.
- Symptomatic treatment.
- Glucocorticoids usually not indicated.

Toxic epidermal necrolysis

Cause and pathogenesis

- Very rare severe cutaneous immunological reaction triggered by:
  - Drugs* (both topical, e.g. antiparasitic dips, and systemic, e.g. antibiotics, antiserum drugs).
  - Infection.
  - Neoplasia.
  - Systemic disease.
  - Idiopathic causes.*
- Overlap occurs between this disease and severe forms of erythema multiforme.

Clinical signs

- Severe cases are rapidly fatal.
- Cutaneous lesions.
  - Lesions can be found on any area of the body but especially the mouth, mucocutaneous junctions and feet.
  - Vesicles, bullae, erosions, ulceration.
- Non-cutaneous lesions.
  - Depression, anorexia, pyrexia.

Differential diagnosis

- Erythema multiforme.
- Burns.
- Contact irritant/allergy.
- Epitheliotrophic lymphoma.
- Systemic lupus erythematosus.

Diagnosis

- History and clinical signs.
- Skin biopsy – full thickness coagulation necrosis of epidermis.

Treatment

- Poor prognosis.
- Identification and treatment of underlying cause where possible.

---

*Reported in the cat.

- Symptomatic and supportive treatment including hospitalisation, fluids, topical and antibiotic therapy, the latter only where there has been no previous inter-reactive drug administration.
- Glucocorticoids may be useful in some cases.

Vasculitis

- Very rare skin disease causing purpura necrosis and ulceration of the extremities.

Cause and pathogenesis

- Both immune and non-immune mechanisms are involved.
- Most cases caused by a type III hypersensitivity reaction which leads to blood vessel damage.
- Causes include:
    - Infection (bacterial, mycobacterial, fungal, viral, protozoal, rickettsial).
    - Malignancy (Fig. 7.17).
    - Connective tissue disease.
    - Drugs.
    - Idiopathic (approximately 50%).

Clinical signs

- No age, sex or breed predisposition.
- Cutaneous lesions.
    - Purpura, haemorrhagic bullae, 'punched out' ulcers found on extremities (Fig. 7.18).
    - Lesions often wedge shaped (Fig. 7.19).
    - Pain variable.

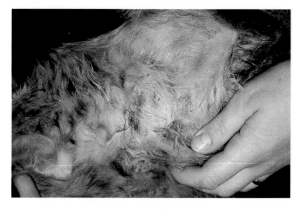

Fig. 7.17 Erythema and necrosis on ventral abdomen of cat with vasculitis due to a liver tumour.

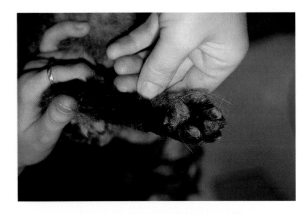

Fig. 7.18 Ulceration of footpads due to vasculitis.

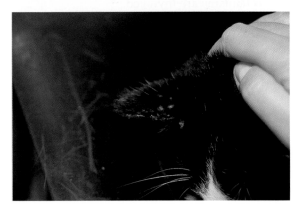

Fig. 7.19 Punched out ulcers on the ear of a cat with vasculitis.

- Non-cutaneous lesions dependent on underlying cause include:
  - ○ Anorexia, lethargy, pyrexia.
  - ○ Oedema of extremities.
  - ○ Polyarthropathy, myopathy.

Differential diagnosis

- Systemic lupus erythematosus.
- Cold agglutinin disease.
- Frostbite.
- Coagulopathy.
- Toxoplasmosis.

Diagnosis

- History and clinical signs.
- Skin biopsy – neutrophilic or lymphocytic vasculitis, often cell poor interface changes and 'faded' follicles.

Treatment

- Identification and treatment of underlying cause.
- Prognosis depends on trigger factors.
- Treatment of vasculitis.
  - Every effort should be made to ensure there is no underlying infective trigger before using immunosuppressive therapy.
  - Prednisolone – 2–4 mg/kg by mouth once daily.
  - Often long term maintenance treatment is required.

Cutaneous drug reactions

- Uncommon cutaneous or mucocutaneous reaction to a drug.

Cause and pathogenesis

- Drugs administered orally, topically, ingested or inhaled.
- Type of reactions.
  - Predictable – dose dependent related to pharmacological action of the drug.
  - Unpredictable – idiosyncratic reaction or drug intolerance.
- Groups of drugs most commonly implicated as causing hypersensitivity-like reactions in the cat:
  - Antibiotics – especially potentiated sulphonamides.
  - Anthelmintics.
  - Vaccines.

Clinical signs

- Many different cutaneous patterns can be associated with drug reactions; these include:
  - Urticaria, angioedema.
  - Erythema multiforme.
  - Toxic epidermal necrolysis.
  - Bullous pemphigoid.
  - Pemphigus foliaceus.
  - Vasculitis.
- Drug reactions can mimic almost any disease.
- Onset of reaction is usually within 2 weeks of the drug administration.
- Resolution usually 10–14 days after withdrawal of drug.

Differential diagnosis

- Almost any other disease.

Diagnosis

- History – an accurate knowledge of any prescribed medication is essential. Drugs can include food additives, supplements, etc., as well as medication given.

- Biopsy – many different patterns, therefore non-diagnostic; necrotic keratinocytes often seen.

Treatment

- Discontinuation of offending drug essential.
- Home cooked diet of single protein and carbohydrate source.
- Symptomatic treatment for clinical signs – fluid therapy in severe cases.
- Avoid chemically related drugs.

Relapsing polychondritis

- Rare immune mediated disease caused by inflammation and destruction of both articular and non-articular cartilaginous structures.

Cause and pathogenesis

- Thought to be an immune mediated attack on type II collagen.
- All reported cases have been either FeLV positive or FIV positive.

Clinical signs

- Affects the ears producing:
  - Acutely painful swollen, erythematous/violaceous pinnae becoming curled and deformed (Fig. 7.20).
- Systemic signs variable.
  - Cats may be quiet, pyrexic and anorexic.

Differential diagnosis

- Trauma.
- Aural haematoma.

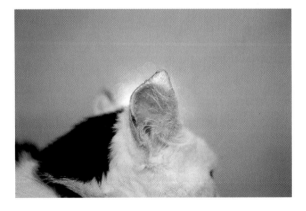

Fig. 7.20 Polychondritis showing deformity of the ear pinna.

Diagnosis

- Clinical signs.
- Biopsy – lymphoplasmacytic inflammation with cartilage necrosis.

Treatment

- Permanent deformity of the pinna occurs whether the cat is treated or not.
- Immunosuppressive therapy with either prednisolone or dapsone – 1 mg/kg by mouth daily – may be effective.

Amyloidosis

- Rare cutaneous manifestation of abnormal extracellular deposition of amyloid.

Cause and pathogenesis

- Deposition of amyloid usually associated with chronic inflammatory disease – especially renal disease.

Clinical signs

- Solitary or grouped dermal or subcutaneous nodules at any site but especially ears.

Differential diagnosis

- Neoplasia.
- Infectious nodular granulomas.
- Sterile nodular granulomas.

Diagnosis

- History – chronic internal disease.
- Clinical signs.
- Skin biopsy – special stains to identify amyloid.

Treatment

- Solitary nodules without internal disease – surgical incision.
- Where associated with systemic disease prognosis guarded.

Alopecia areata

Cause and pathogenesis

- Thought to be immunological attack of hair bulb by lymphocytes leading to non-inflammatory hair loss.

Clinical signs

- No sex, breed, age predilection.
- Focal or multifocal patches of asymptomatic non-inflammatory alopecia – especially on head, neck, trunk.
- Chronic lesions can become hyperpigmented.
- Non-pruritic.

Differential diagnosis

- Drug eruption.
- Demodicosis.
- Dermatophytosis.
- Psychogenic alopecia.
- Pseudopelade.

Diagnosis

- History and clinical signs.
- Trichography – 'exclamation point' hairs – tapered ends, dystrophic hairs.
- Skin biopsy – peribulbar lymphocytes 'swarm of bees' – multiple biopsies usually required.

Treatment

- Most cases recover spontaneously in 6 months to 2 years.
- Glucocorticoid treatment – topical or systemic steroids give variable benefits.

Pseudopelade

Cause and pathogenesis

- Very rare acquired alopecia characterised by lymphocyte attack of follicular isthmus, leading to non-inflammatory hair loss.

Clinical signs

- No sex, breed, age predilection.
- Non-inflammatory alopecia of ventrum and legs, can be localised or generalised.
- Non-pruritic.
- Onychomadesis.

Differential diagnosis

- Drug eruption.
- Demodicosis.
- Dermatophytosis.

- Psychogenic alopecia.
- Alopecia areata.

Diagnosis

- History and clinical signs.
- Trichography – dystrophic hairs are not seen.
- Skin biopsy – lymphocyte infiltration mid follicle, chronically damaged hairs are atrophic.

Treatment

- Variable response to therapy.
- Immunosuppressive therapy with glucocorticoids may be useful.

Chapter 8

Endocrine and Metabolic Skin Diseases

Hyperadrenocorticism (feline Cushing's syndrome)

- A rare disease in the cat caused by increased levels of circulating cortisol.
- Management of other concurrent problems such as respiratory infections, diabetes, etc., is more easily achieved once the hyperadrenocorticism is controlled.

Cause and pathogenesis

Naturally occurring hyperadrenocorticism

- Pituitary dependent hyperadrenocorticism (80% of naturally occurring cases).
  - ○ Seen as a bilateral adrenocortical hyperplasia due to pituitary adenoma or adenocarcinoma.
  - ○ Defective negative feedback of adrenocorticotrophic hormone (ACTH) at level of hypothalamus.
- Adrenal dependent hyperadrenocorticism.
  - ○ Adrenocortical neoplasia due to a functional adenoma or adenocarcinoma.

Iatrogenic hyperadrenocorticism

- Chronic overuse of steroids by injection or tablet.
- Rare in the cat due to high steroid tolerance.

Clinical signs

Naturally occurring hyperadrenocorticism

- Middle–old age cat, females predisposed.
- No breed predisposition.
- Non-cutaneous signs:
  - ○ General:
    Polydipsia, polyuria.
    Polyphagia.
    Depression.
    Anorexia, weight loss.

90% of cats are prediabetic or overtly diabetic (due to corticosteroid induced insulin antagonism).

○ Neuromuscular signs:
Muscle atrophy, pot-bellied appearance (Fig. 8.1)

○ Respiratory signs:
Recurrent respiratory infections.

• Cutaneous signs (in decreasing order of frequency):

○ Alopecia – partial or complete, involving dorsum, flanks or ventrum (Fig. 8.2).

○ Thin/fragile skin, often tears with routine handling (Fig. 8.3).

○ Easy bruising (Fig. 8.4).

○ Poor hair coat/seborrhoea.

○ Secondary infection with bacteria, yeast or *Demodex* – response to therapy is poor in these cases unless hyperadrenocorticism is treated concurrently.

○ Comedones.

○ Hyperpigmentation.

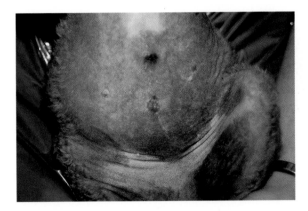

Fig. 8.1 Pot-bellied appearance in naturally occurring hyperadrenocorticism.

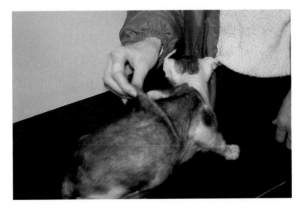

Fig. 8.2 Thin alopecic skin on dorsum and flanks in cat with hyperadrenocorticism.

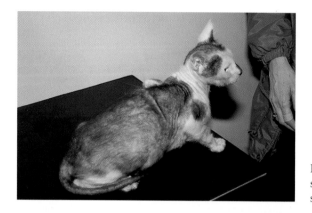

Fig. 8.3 Same cat as Fig. 8.2 – skin remains tented after release, showing lack of elasticity.

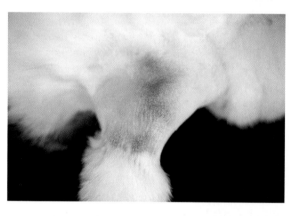

Fig. 8.4 Bruising at the site of blood sampling in cat with hyperadrenocorticism.

Iatrogenic hyperadrenocorticism

- Any age, sex or breed.
- Clinical signs similar to naturally occurring disease except in addition:
  - Medial curling of ear tips.

Differential diagnosis

- Cutaneous lesions especially where alopecia is present.
  - Traumatic alopecia (allergy, psychogenic alopecia, parasites, etc.).
  - Diabetes mellitus.
  - Hyperthyroidism.
  - Cutaneous asthenia.
  - Pancreatic paraneoplastic alopecia.
  - Acquired skin fragility.

Diagnosis

- History and clinical signs.
- No consistent findings on haematology or biochemistry other than hyperglycaemia.

- ○ Hypercholesterolaemia ~50%.
- ○ Elevations of serum alanine aminotransferase (ALT) ~40%.
- ○ Elevations in serum alkaline phosphatase (SAP) ~20%.
- Urine sample glycosuria where concurrent diabetes mellitus.
- Radiography – hepatomegaly.
- Other imaging techniques include ultrasound, computer tomography to identify adrenal or pituitary masses.
- Skin biopsy – decreased dermal collagen, no other specific changes.

Adrenal function tests

- These are poorly described. Always consult your laboratory for advice before performing these tests in the cat.
- ACTH stimulation test – many different protocols have been described.
  - ○ Protocol – two separate cortisol peaks are seen in the cat after stimulation; therefore blood samples are taken to measure cortisol levels at time 0, then 1 and 2 hours after the intravenous administration of 125 µg synthacthen.
  - ○ Most cats with hyperadrenocorticism show an exaggerated response to ACTH.
- Low dose dexamethasone suppression test – not well standardised in the cat.
  - ○ Dexamethasone at a dose of 0.01–0.015 mg/kg intravenously will often not suppress cortisol in normal cats. Essentially this screening test is a high dose suppression test.
  - ○ Protocol – blood samples are taken to measure cortisol levels at time 0 and 8 hours after the intravenous administration of 0.1 mg/kg dexamethasone.
  - ○ Cortisol levels in most cats with hyperadrenocorticism fail to suppress.
- Combined test.
  - ○ Protocol – collect a baseline blood sample for serum cortisol. Administer a high dose of dexamethasone (0.1 mg/kg intravenously). Collect a post dexamethasone sample for serum cortisol after 2 hours. At the same time administer 125 µg synthacthen intravenously. Collect a third sample for cortisol estimation a further 1 hour later.
  - ○ Cortisol levels in cats with hyperadrenocorticism usually do not suppress after dexamethasone administration and overstimulate after synthacthen.

Treatment of naturally occurring disease

Medical therapy

- A poor response has been recorded to any medical therapy. Surgical management is preferable. However, where surgery is impossible then:
  - ○ Mitotane is of no value in therapy in the cat.
  - ○ Metyrapone – blocks adrenal synthesis of steroids. Dosage 250–500 mg per cat per day by mouth is the most promising of all medical therapies. The response to treatment is monitored by a reduction in ACTH stimulation and improvement in clinical signs.

○ Ketoconazole – interferes with adrenal steroid synthesis in dogs but does not cause same effect in the cat and has thus no benefit in this disease. Dosage 10–15 mg/kg by mouth twice daily.
○ The use of other drugs such as bromocriptine, cyproheptadine and selegiline has not been documented in the cat.

Surgical therapy

- Pituitary dependent disease – bilateral adrenalectomy followed by lifelong therapy for hypoadrenocorticism.
- Adrenal neoplasia – removal of neoplastic adrenal gland (usually unilateral) is curative.

Radiotherapy

- Has been used with partial success to treat some cats with pituitary dependent disease. Limited availability.

Hypothyroidism

- Very rare endocrine skin disease in the cat.

Cause and pathogenesis

Adult onset hypothyroidism

- Spontaneously occurring – very rare disease.
- Iatrogenic disease – secondary to radioactive iodine therapy or thyroidectomy for hyperthyroidism.

Congenital hypothyroidism

- Seen in young kittens.
- Caused by a variety of mechanisms all of which are thought to be inherited as an autosomal recessive trait.
  ○ Thyroid gland agenesis/dysgenesis.
  ○ Dyshormonogenesis.
  ○ Impaired organification of iodides (domestic short haired cats and Abyssinians).
  ○ Inability of the gland to respond to thyroid stimulating hormone.

Clinical signs

Adult onset – spontaneously occurring

- Non-cutaneous signs:
  ○ Lethargy, obesity, heat seeking.

- Cutaneous signs:
  - Dry dull brittle hair coat.
  - Myxoedema – cool puffy skin.
  - Variable pigment changes to skin and coat.
  - Seborrhoea generalised.
  - Delayed wound healing – poor hair regrowth after clipping.
  - Alopecia not normally a feature – some cats may lose hair from their ears.

Adult onset – iatrogenic

- Non-cutaneous signs:
  - Initial lethargy but usually short lived.
  - No changes in body weight or appetite.
- Cutaneous signs:
  - Generalised seborrhoea.
  - Dorsal matting due to reduced grooming activity.
  - Alopecia of pressure points, pinnae, dorsal and lateral tail base region.

Congenital hypothyroidism

- Very rare – kittens 4 weeks of age.
- Often kittens will die at an early age before hypothyroidism is suspected.
- Non-cutaneous signs:
  - Lethargic and mentally dull.
  - Decreased rate of growth, stunted.
  - Disproportionate dwarfs.
  - Short broad head, enlarged skull, shortened limbs, retained deciduous teeth, short round body, small ears.
- Cutaneous signs:
  - Hair coat fine due to reduction in primary hairs – alopecia rare.
  - Seborrhoea.
  - Thickened skin.

Differential diagnosis

- Traumatic alopecia, e.g. due to allergy, ectoparasites, psychogenic.
- Dermatophytosis.
- Demodicosis.
- Hyperadrenocorticism.
- Hyperthyroidism.

Diagnosis

- History and clinical signs.
- Haematology and biochemistry not fully evaluated as a diagnostic aid.
  - Non-specific but inconsistent changes include normochromic, normocytic, non-regenerative anaemia and hypercholesterolaemia.
- Thyroid function tests:

○ Basal levels of total thyroxine (TT_4), free thyroxine (FT_4), total triiodothyronine (TT_3), and free triiodothyronine (FT_3) – can be misleading. For congenital hypothyroidism by 4 weeks of age TT_4 should be within the range 52–72 nmol/l, for a normal cat.
Non-thyroidal illness (euthyroid sick syndrome) and drug therapy (steroids, barbiturates) can influence these tests.
○ TSH stimulation tests – superior to basal thyroid levels. Contact laboratory for advice before performing the test.
Protocol – measure T_4 level before and 6–7 hours after administration of 0.5–1.0 IU/kg of bovine TSH.
Healthy cats double or treble their levels; hypothyroid cats show little or no response.
○ TRH stimulation test – most reliable test for diagnosis of hypothyroidism in the cat.
Measure T_4 levels before and 4 hours after the slow (may induce vomiting) intravenous injection of 100 μg of TRH.
Healthy cats demonstrate a 50–100% rise in T_4; hypothyroid cats fail to respond.
○ Thyroid biopsy – not useful in practice.

Treatment

- Lifetime treatment required in all cases.
- Supplementation.
  ○ Levothyroxine (T_4) (Soloxine, Vet-2-Vet).
  Orally 0.05–0.2 mg per cat once daily.
  The response to therapy depends on the form of disease.
  Congenital hypothyroidism is often poorly responsive.
  With acquired hypothyroidism an excellent response can be expected:
  Lethargy improves, often within days.
  Cutaneous lesions can take up to 6 weeks to respond.
  ○ Liothyronine (T_3) supplementation is rarely indicated.

Hyperthyroidism

- Very common endocrine disorder caused by over production of thyroid hormone thyroxine (T_4) and triiodothyronine (T_3).

Cause and pathogenesis

- Solitary thyroid adenoma or multinodular adenomatous hyperplasia of the thyroid.
- Carcinomas of the gland are rare.
- Clinical signs are caused by the resulting acceleration in basal metabolic rate.

Clinical signs

- Age incidence 6–20 years, average age 12 years.
- No breed or sex predilection.
- Onset of signs insidious.
- 95% of cats have a palpable enlarged cervical mass (Fig. 8.5).
- Non-cutaneous signs:
  - Weight loss (Fig. 8.6).
  - Polyphagia.
  - Polydipsia.
  - Diarrhoea and vomiting.
  - Hyperactivity.
  - Tachycardia.
  - Respiratory abnormalities.
  - Occasionally lethargy, weakness and inappetence.
- Cutaneous signs seen in about 30–40% of cases:
  - Excessive shedding of hair coat, easily epilated.

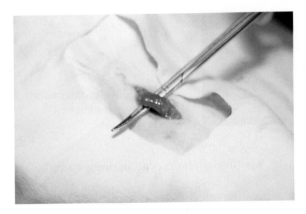

Fig. 8.5 Enlarged thyroid gland – palpable in the conscious cat.

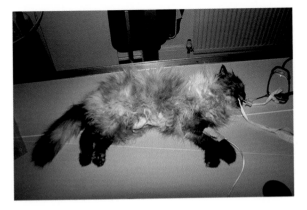

Fig. 8.6 Severe weight loss in an untreated hyperthyroid cat.

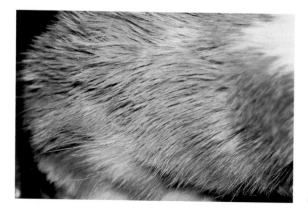

Fig. 8.7 Generalised seborrhoea oleosa in a hyperthyroid cat.

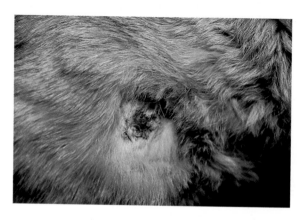

Fig. 8.8 Acute moist dermatitis due to overgrooming in a hyperthyroid cat.

○ Seborrhoea oleosa leading to matting of hair coat in long-haired cats (Fig. 8.7).
○ Focal, often bilaterally symmetrical alopecia (usually flanks) due to over-grooming. In severe cases, self-inflicted trauma can occur (Fig. 8.8).
○ Increased claw growth.

Differential diagnosis

- Hyperadrenocorticism.
- Allergy (food, fleas, atopy).*
- Dermatophytosis.*
- Psychogenic alopecia.

Diagnosis

- History and clinical signs – especially palpable thyroid nodule.
- Haematology limited diagnostically.

---

*Can occur concurrently exacerbated by hyperthyroid state.

- Biochemistry – increases seen in serum alkaline phosphatase (SAP), lactate dehydrogenase (LDH), alanine aminotransferase (ALT) and aspartate transaminase (AST).

Thyroid function tests
- Elevations in basal levels of total T_4 (TT_4) and total T_3 (TT_3).
  - ○ False negative reaction – depression of elevated levels can occur due to: Euthyroid sick state, e.g. concurrent renal disease, diabetes.
    Concurrent therapy – especially long acting steroids (e.g. methyl prednisolone acetate) and hormones (e.g. megoestrol acetate).
    Sedation undertaken where cat is difficult to blood sample.
    Early stages of the disease – retest 6–8 weeks later.
  - ○ False positive reaction – due to overlap with normal cats.
- T_3 suppression test.
  - ○ 15–25 µg of liothyronine given orally every 8 hours for seven doses. TT_4 and free T_4 (FT_4) levels are measured before drug administration and 2–4 hours after the last dose.
  - ○ Hyperthyroid cats show no change in their TT_4 or FT_4 levels.
  - ○ Normal cats show a 50% depression in TT_4 and FT_4.
- TSH stimulation test.
  - ○ 0.5 IU/kg intravenous injection of bovine TSH.
  - ○ Bloods taken at 0 and 6 hours.
  - ○ Euthyroid cats show a 100% increase in TT_4; hyperthyroid cats minimal or no increase.
- TRH stimulation test.
  - ○ 0.1 mg/kg TRH by slow intravenous injection.
  - ○ Bloods taken at 0 and 4 hours.
  - ○ Euthyroid cats show a greater than 60% increase in TT_4.
  - ○ Hyperthyroid cats show less than 50% increase in TT_4 levels.

Radionuclide imaging
- Thyroid scanning is undertaken after the intravenous administration of a suitable radionuclide, e.g. technetium-99M (pertechnetate). Radionuclide is concentrated in a hyperactive gland.

Treatment
- Surgical excision (see further reading list for suitable surgical texts for details of thyroidectomy).
  - ○ Advantages:
    Inexpensive.
    Accessible surgery that can be performed in a normal practice.
  - ○ Disadvantages:
    Anaesthetic risk, especially if tachycardia, or renal dysfunction.
    Induction of thyrotoxic crisis.

Iatrogenic hypoparathyroidism.
Iatrogenic hypothyroidism.
Incomplete removal and recurrence.
Risk of damage to recurrent laryngeal nerve.
- Oral antithyroid drugs:
  - ○ Carbimazole (Neo-mercazole, Nicholas) 5 mg per cat by mouth three times daily.
  - ○ Methimazole (not available in the UK).
  - ○ Propanolol may be used to treat tachycardia.
  - ○ Advantages:
    Inexpensive and efficacious.
    Outpatient basis.
  - ○ Disadvantages:
    Side effects of medication include anorexia, vomiting, anaemia and thrombocytopaenia.
    Many hyperthyroid cats are difficult to medicate with oral drugs.
    Iatrogenic hypothyroidism.
    Monitoring necessary, TT_4 and FT_4 levels taken every 2 weeks during induction period and every 3 months during maintenance.
- Radioactive iodine.
  - ○ Advantages:
    Single treatment only.
    No anaesthetic or surgery.
    Highly efficacious.
  - ○ Disadvantages:
    Sophisticated facilities needed including hospitalisation and isolation cages.
    Expensive.
    Risk of medication to human contacts.
    Iatrogenic hypothyroidism.
    Re-treatment necessary in 20–30% of cats.

Pituitary dwarfism

- Hereditary hypopituitarism leading to proportionate dwarfism.

Cause and pathogenesis

- Clinical signs principally of growth hormone deficiency; also thyroidal, adrenocortical and gonadal hormones affected.

Clinical signs

- Kittens are normal for the first 2–3 months, then fail to grow.
- Cutaneous signs:

- ○ Mild signs of seborrhoea are often the only change noted.
- ○ Alopecia, coat and pigmentation are rare.
- Non-cutaneous signs:
  - ○ Mental dullness.
  - ○ Musculoskeletal – stunted growth, square chunky contour, delayed growth plate closure.
  - ○ Reproduction – failure to cycle, testicular atrophy.
  - ○ Reduced life expectancy.
  - ○ Delayed eruption of permanent teeth.

Differential diagnosis

- Hypothyroidism.
- Cardiovascular disease.
- Congenital hepatic disease (portosystemic shunts).
- Hypoadrenocorticism.

Diagnosis

- History and clinical signs – especially compared to litter mates.
- Laboratory tests to rule out primary thyroid and adrenocortical disease.
- Radiography – delayed closure of long bones, delayed eruption of permanent teeth.
- Basal growth hormone levels not reliable.
- Dynamic function tests:
  - ○ Inadequate release of growth hormone is demonstrated by either clonidine, xylazine or growth hormone releasing hormone stimulation tests.
  - ○ These are poorly documented in the cat, and are not widely available.
  - ○ Consult your local laboratory for details.
- Insulin-like growth factor-1 (IGF-1).
  - ○ A single basal sample can be used to assess pituitary function indirectly.
  - ○ Healthy dogs and cats 200–800 ng/ml.
  - ○ Growth hormone deficiency cats <50 ng/ml.
  - ○ Test only available through special laboratories.

Treatment

- Growth hormone replacement therapy with porcine or bovine growth hormone.
  - ○ Risks of hypersensitivity and diabetes mellitus.
- Thyroid, steroid replacement therapy if appropriate.

Acromegaly

- Rare disease caused by overproduction of growth hormone in the mature cat usually presents as poorly controlled diabetes mellitus.

Cause and pathogenesis

- Hypersecretion of growth hormone in the mature animal leads to overgrowth of connective tissue, bones and viscera.
- Pituitary neoplasia most common cause of acromegaly in the cat due to a functional growth-hormone-secreting adenoma/adenocarcinoma of anterior pituitary gland.
- Unlike the dog, progestogens do not stimulate excessive growth hormone secretion in the cat.

Clinical signs

- Non-cutaneous signs
  - Increased size of extremities, paws and skull.
  - Polyuria, polydipsia (due to poorly controlled concurrent diabetes mellitus).
  - Prognathism, widening of interdental spaces.
  - Neurological signs may be present (15%).
  - Inspiratory stridor – rare finding in the cat compared to dog.
  - Renal failure common (50%).
  - Cardiac failure – common (40%).
  - Arthropathy (40%).
- Cutaneous signs
  - Myxoedema, excessive skin folds.

Differential diagnosis

- Hyperadrenocorticism.
- Hypothyroidism.
- Diabetes mellitus.

Diagnosis

- History and clinical signs.
- Biochemistry – elevations of glucose, serum alkaline phosphatase, alanine aminotransferase.
- Skin biopsy – increase in collagen and mucin in dermis, myxoedema may be present.
- Measurement of growth hormone levels – demonstration of high circulating levels.
  - Limited availability of the assay.
- Insulin-like growth factor-1 (IGF-1)
  - A single basal sample can be used to assess pituitary function indirectly.
  - Healthy dogs and cats 200–800 ng/ml.
  - Acromegaly cats >1000 ng/ml.
  - Test only available through special laboratories.

- Diagnostic imaging with computer tomography (CT) or magnetic resonance imaging (MRI).

Treatment

- Pituitary neoplasia.
  - Medical treatment with bromocriptine, octreotide is unrewarding.
  - Surgical treatment – hypophysectomy or pituitary radiation through referral centre are possible options.

Pancreatic paraneoplastic alopecia

- Cutaneous manifestation of pancreatic neoplasia.

Cause and pathogenesis

- Most reported cases have had a pancreatic carcinoma of either the acinar cell or pancreatic duct origin. Metastasis to liver common.

Clinical signs

- Old cats (9–16 years old).
- No breed or sex predilection.
- Cutaneous signs
  - Acute onset of rapidly progressive alopecia involving the ventrum and legs.
  - Hair is easily epilated in non-alopecic areas.
  - Alopecic skin often smooth and 'glistening'.
  - Pruritus usually minimal.
  - Painful footpads, often thin, occasionally fissured.
- Non-cutaneous signs
  - Inappetence, lethargy.
  - Weight loss.

Differential diagnosis

- Hyperadrenocorticism.
- Cutaneous fragility syndrome.
- Telogen defluxion.
- Traumatic alopecia (allergy, ectoparasites, psychogenic).
- Metabolic epidermal necrosis.

Diagnosis

- History and clinical signs.
- Skin biopsy – exfoliation of stratum corneum, laminated orthokeratosis alternating with focal parakeratosis, follicular atrophy.
- Diagnostic rule-outs, i.e. haematology, biochemistry, ACTH, usually unremarkable.
- Abdominal diagnostic imaging – radiographs, ultrasounds to look for neoplasia.
- Exploratory laparotomy.

Treatment

- None currently available.
- Grave prognosis, cats deteriorate rapidly and die.

Metabolic epidermal necrosis

- Cutaneous manifestation of pancreatic disease. Overlap may occur between this disease and pancreatic paraneoplastic alopecia.

Cause and pathogenesis

- Very rare disease – recorded cases to date have been attributed to pancreatic carcinomas.

Clinical signs

- Old cats, no breed or age predilection.
- Cutaneous signs
  - Alopecia of axilla and legs.
  - Thickened seborrhoeic skin.
  - Erythema and exudation.
  - Footpad hyperkeratosis is an inconsistent finding.
- Non-cutaneous signs
  - Anorexia, lethargy.

Differential diagnosis

- As pancreatic paraneoplastic alopecia (PPA).

Diagnosis

- History and clinical signs.
- Diagnostic rule-out as PPA.

- Skin biopsy – parakeratosis, oedema of upper epidermis, irregular epidermal hyperplasia (red, white and blue).
- Abdominal diagnostic imaging – radiographs, ultrasounds to look for neoplasia.
- Exploratory laparotomy.

Treatment

- Unsuccessful.

Xanthoma

Cause and pathogenesis

- Granulomatous lesions associated with abnormalities in lipid metabolism including:
  - Hereditary hyperlipoproteinaemia.
  - Diabetes mellitus (naturally occurring and drug induced).
  - Idiopathic disease.

Clinical signs

- Cutaneous signs:
  - Lesions typically affect head, extremities and bony prominences.
  - Multiple white or yellow papules, nodules or plaques.
  - Surrounding skin erythematous.
  - Often painful and pruritic.
- Non-cutaneous signs:
  - Associated with concurrent diabetes or hyperlipoproteinaemia.

Differential diagnosis

- Eosinophilic granuloma complex.
- Cutaneous neoplasia (lymphoma, mast cell tumour).
- Cutaneous horn.
- Callus.
- Metastatic calcification – chronic renal disease.

Diagnosis

- History and clinical signs.
- Skin biopsy – multinucleate giant cells, foamy macrophages.
- Investigation of underlying fault in lipid metabolism, including biochemistry and glucose levels.

Treatment

- Medical treatment.
  - Therapy of underlying problem will result in spontaneous resolution of lesions, i.e. stabilisation of diabetes mellitus, high fibre/low fat diet in idiopathic cases.
- Surgical treatment.
  - Unsuccessful, only results in recurrence of lesions.

Chapter 9

Alopecia

- Alopecia has been classified based on the scheme suggested for alopecia in the dog by Professor Robert Dunstan.
- Follicular dystrophy.
  - ○ Congenital.
    Congenital hypotrichosis.
    Pili torti.
  - ○ Acquired.
    Anagen defluxion.
- Hair cycle abnormalities.
  - ○ Hyperadrenocorticism (see Chapter 8).
  - ○ Feline acquired symmetrical alopecia.
  - ○ Telogen defluxion.
  - ○ Pancreatic paraneoplastic alopecia (see Chapter 8).
  - ○ Feline pinnal alopecia.
- Traumatic alopecia.
  - ○ Loss of normal hair.
  - ○ Loss of abnormal hair.
- Scarring alopecia.
  - ○ Primary.
  - ○ Secondary.

FOLLICULAR DYSTROPHY

- Abnormal hairs or follicles are formed due to the abnormal development or growth of the hair. This often leads to alopecia.
- Can be congenital or acquired.

CONGENITAL FOLLICULAR DYSTROPHIES

Congenital hypotrichosis

Cause and pathogenesis

- Cats with congenital hypotrichosis are born without hair or else lose it within the first 4 weeks of life.

- Some animals have only lack of hair follicles; others have additional ectodermal defects.

Clinical signs

- Predisposed breeds include Birman, Burmese, Devon Rex (Fig. 9.1) and Siamese.
- Cats can be born without any hair or with only fine downy hair that is lost within a few weeks (Fig. 9.2).
- In some cases whiskers, claws or papillae on the tongue can be affected.

Differential diagnosis

- Demodicosis.
- Nutritional deficiencies.

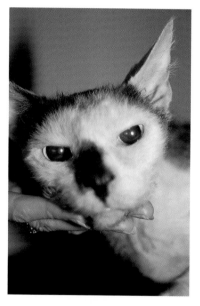

Fig. 9.1 Congenital hypotrichosis in a Devon Rex cross cat.

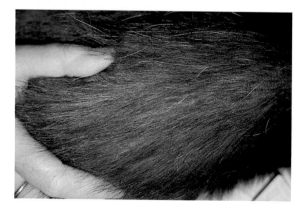

Fig. 9.2 Follicular dystrophy in a domestic short haired grey cat.

- Dermatophytosis.
- Pili torti.

Diagnosis

- History and clinical signs.
- Diagnostic rule-outs, e.g. skin scrapings, fungal culture.
- Skin biopsy – changes range from presence of dystrophic hair follicles to complete lack of follicles, often with similar changes in the adnexal glands.

Treatment

- None.

Pili torti

Cause and pathogenesis

- Rare disease caused by curvature of the hair follicle leading to a flattening and rotation of the hair shaft.

Clinical signs

- Young kittens affected.
- Generalised hair loss by 10 days of age.
- Periocular and pedal dermatitis plus paronychia.

Differential diagnosis

- As congenital hypotrichosis.

Diagnosis

- History and clinical signs.
- Trichography – all secondary hairs flattened and rotated.
- Skin biopsy – not diagnostic; follicular hyperkeratosis and occasional cystic dilatation noted.

Treatment

- None.

ACQUIRED FOLLICULAR DYSTROPHY

Anagen defluxion

Cause and pathogenesis

- Caused by:
  - Antimitotic drugs – cancer, chemotherapy (Fig. 9.3).
  - Infectious disease – FeLV, FIV, FIP.

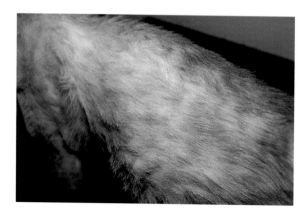

Fig. 9.3 Anagen defluxion causing diffuse hair loss in a cat on chemotherapy.

- ○ Endocrine disease – diabetes mellitus.
- ○ Metabolic disease.
- Anagen growth phase is temporarily halted leading to abnormalities of the hair.
- Hair is lost within days of insult as dystrophic change is incompatible with normal hair growth.

Clinical signs

- Diffuse hair loss usually on dorsum, flanks and ventrum.

Diagnosis

- History – of previous insult to hair cycle.
- Clinical signs.
- Skin biopsy – useful before hair is lost completely.

Treatment

- None.
- Treatment of underlying insult where possible to prevent recurrence.

HAIR CYCLE ABNORMALITIES

Hyperadrenocorticism (see Chapter 8)

Feline acquired symmetrical alopecia

- A very rare bilaterally symmetrical alopecia of unknown origin.
- Originally called feline endocrine alopecia.
- No true hormonal cause has been identified for this disease.

Cause and pathogenesis

- Thyroid function tests in these cats are normal. However, they may have a decreased thyroid reserve based on the fact many respond to thyroid supplementation with liothyronine.
- Response to thyroxine may be non-specific due to psychological factors rather than a deficiency state.

Clinical signs

- No breed predilection.
- Age range 2–12 years.
- Bilaterally symmetrical alopecia.
- Hair can be easily epilated.
- Affected areas – anogenital, proximal tail, caudomedial thighs and ventral abdominal skin.
- Non-pruritic.

Differential diagnosis

Traumatic alopecia

- Ectoparasites (fleas, *Cheyletiella*, *Otodectes*, lice, *Demodex*).
- Allergy (atopy, food).
- Psychogenic alopecia.
- Dermatophytosis.

Non-pruritic alopecia

- Hypothyroidism (very rare).
- Hyperadrenocorticism (very rare).
- Telogen defluxion.
- Anagen defluxion.

Diagnosis

- History and clinical signs.
- Diagnostic rule-out, e.g. skin scrapings, food trial, ectoparasite control.
- Routine blood samples including thyroid and adrenal function tests are normal.
- Trichography – distal hair tips intact and pointed, bulb telogenized.
- Use of Elizabethan collar – if cats are licking out hair the coat will grow back with the use of a collar.
- Skin biopsy – hair telogenized.

Treatment

- *As this is a benign disease the author would consider the side effects of therapy outweigh the benefits.*

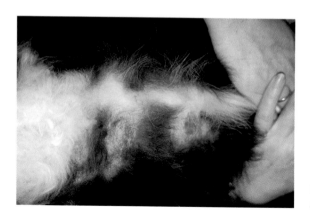

Fig. 9.4 Mammary hyperplasia after therapy with progestagens.

- *Therapy should only be considered once a diagnosis has been made. Empirical therapy for alopecia is not appropriate.*
- Drugs that have been used:
  - ○ Liothyronine – 20 μg per cat orally twice daily may be increased to 50 μg/cat for 12 weeks.
    Side effects – cardiac arrhythmias.
  - ○ Androgen/oestrogen therapy – intramuscular injections of testosterone 12.5 mg total testosterone per cat with oestradiol 0.5 mg per cat. Injections of both are given on two occasions 6 weeks apart. Oestradiol is unlicensed for use in the cat.
    Side effects – oestrous in females, urine spraying and aggressiveness in males. Hepatobiliary, renal and cardiac disease in cases of overdosage.
  - ○ Progestagens – megoestrol acetate orally 2.5–5.0 mg per cat once every other day until hair regrows, then a maintenance dose of 2.5–5.0 mg per cat every 1–2 weeks, or intramuscular injection of medroxyprogesterone acetate 50–175 mg per cat two injections given 6 weeks apart.
    Side effects – adrenal suppression, diabetes mellitus, mammary gland fibroadenomatous hyperplasia which can progress to neoplasia (Fig. 9.4).

Telogen defluxion

Cause and pathogenesis

- Abrupt stressful circumstance, e.g. pyrexia, systemic illness, pregnancy, surgery, leads to cessation of anagen phase of cycle.
- Hairs synchronised in catagen then telogen to be lost 1–3 months after initial insult.

Clinical signs

- Sudden and widespread hair loss (Fig. 9.5).

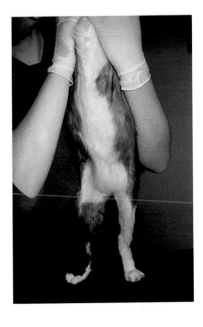

Fig. 9.5 Telogen defluxion in a heavily pregnant queen.

Diagnosis

- History and clinical signs.
- Skin biopsy – rarely diagnostic.

Treatment

- Therapy of underlying disease.
- Hair will grow back without therapy if underlying problem is resolved.

Pancreatic paraneoplastic alopecia

- See Chapter 8.

Feline pinnal alopecia

Cause and pathogenesis

- Periodic alopecia of the ears of unknown cause.

Clinical signs

- Siamese predisposed (Fig. 9.6).
- Alopecia typically bilateral, may be patchy or more extensive.
- Hair will spontaneously regrow after several months.

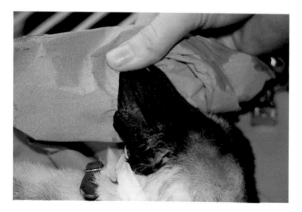

Fig. 9.6 Patchy alopecia on the ear of a Siamese.

Differential diagnosis

- As congenital hypotrichosis.

Diagnosis

- History and clinical signs.
- Diagnostic rule-outs, e.g. skin scrapings, trichography.

Treatment

- Unnecessary as hair will regrow after several months.

TRAUMATIC ALOPECIA

Cause and pathogenesis

- Cats are often secret groomers and due to their fastidious nature overgrooming of normal hair or normal grooming of abnormal hair can produce areas of alopecia, as hair is either nibbled short or else pulled out.

Loss of normal hairs through overgrooming

- Any cause of overgrooming can lead to traumatic hair loss including:
  - Ectoparasites – fleas (Fig. 9.7), *Cheyletiella*, *Otodectes*, lice, *Demodex*.
  - Allergy – atopy (Fig. 9.8), food.
  - Psychogenic alopecia.
  - Dermatophytosis.
  - Hyperthyroidism.
  - Paraneoplastic pruritus.
  - Localised pain, e.g. abdominal or orthopaedic pain.
  - Seborrhoeic dermatitis.

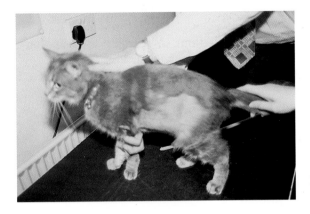

Fig. 9.7 Flank alopecia
secondary to flea allergy.

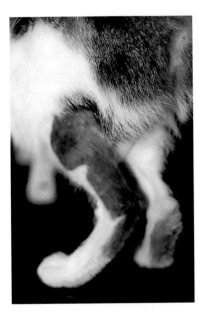

Fig. 9.8 Alopecia on lower legs in a cat with
atopy.

Loss of hairs with shaft abnormalities

- Hairs themselves are abnormal.
- The fault can be induced by damage to the hair by excessive brushing/
  grooming, harsh chemicals, heat, UV radiation, e.g. acquired trichorrhexis
  nodosa leading to subsequent hair loss.
- The fault can be hereditary, e.g. shaft disorder of Abyssinian cats, hereditary
  trichorrhexis nodosa.

Concurrent loss of normal and abnormal hair

- Overgrooming of normal hair and normal grooming of abnormal hair can be
  present concurrently.

Clinical signs

- Alopecia can be complete if the hair is pulled out, or partial if the hairs have been barbered off to give the impression of extensive hair loss.
- Patterns of alopecia are variable and are not specific to any one disease:
  - Bilaterally symmetrical flank alopecia.
  - Ventral abdominal alopecia (Fig. 9.9).
  - Alopecia of caudomedial thighs.
  - Alopecia of lower extremities.
  - Diffuse generalised hair loss (Fig. 9.10).
- These patterns can occur concurrently and also in combination with components of the eosinophilic granuloma complex (see Chapter 17).
- Primary lesions are not usually present.

Differential diagnosis

- Hyperadrenocorticism.
- Hypothyroidism.
- Telogen defluxion.

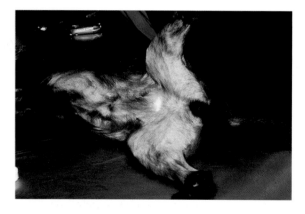

Fig. 9.9 Ventral alopecia secondary to flea allergy.

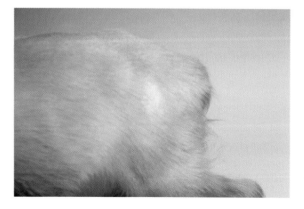

Fig. 9.10 Diffuse hair loss on dorsum secondary to *Cheyletiella*.

- Paraneoplastic alopecia.
- Feline acquired symmetrical alopecia.

Diagnosis

- History and clinical signs.
- Diagnostic rule-out for non-traumatic alopecia.
- Trichography.
  - ○ Loss of normal hairs – bulbs of both anogen and telogen hairs, shafts normal but hair tips barbered, suggesting overgrooming.
  - ○ Loss of abnormal hairs.
    Trichorrhexis nodosa – bulbs and tips as normal hairs, shafts have small bead-like swellings associated with loss of cuticle. Nodular areas of cortical splitting resemble two ends of a brush pushed together (Fig. 9.11).
    Shaft disorders of Abyssinian cats – whiskers and primary hairs only.
    Onion shaped swelling normally seen on the shaft or hair tips.

Treatment

- Identification of underlying cause of pruritus/overgrooming essential where normal hair is lost.
- Hereditary disorders – no treatment has been described.

SCARRING ALOPECIA

- Destruction/distortion of hair follicles.

Primary scarring alopecia

- Folliculitis – inflammatory reactions directed against hair follicles or organisms in lumen caused by infectious or immunological mechanisms including:

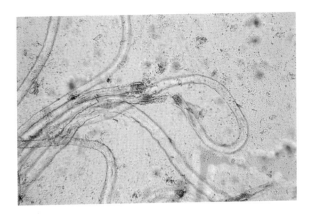

Fig. 9.11 Trichorrhexis nodosa secondary to flea allergy.

- ○ Bacteria – e.g. *Staphylococcus*.
- ○ Dermatophytes – *Microsporum canis*.
- ○ *Demodex cati.*
- ○ Pemphigus complex.

Secondary scarring alopecia

- Hair follicles not primary target – damaged as a bystander.
    - ○ Infarcted hairs, e.g. vasculitis.
    - ○ Perifollicular damage above hair bulb, e.g. sebaceous adenitis.
    - ○ Severe generalised cutaneous damage, e.g. burns.

Chapter 10

Congenital and Hereditary Diseases

DISORDERS OF EPITHELIAL FORMATION

Primary seborrhoea

Cause and pathogenesis

- A very rare disease in the cat.
- Defined as an inherited disorder of keratinisation or cornification.
- The epidermis, follicular epithelium, hair cuticle and the claw can all be involved.
- In most cats seborrhoea is secondary to an underlying disease; every effort should be made to identify this before a diagnosis of primary seborrhoea is made.
- Often clinical signs can be quite mild due to the fastidious grooming behaviour of the cat.

Clinical signs

- Predisposed breed – Persian.
- Identified as an autosomal recessive mode of inheritance.
- Age of onset
  - Severe cases – young kittens by 2–3 days of age.
  - Mild cases – 6 weeks of age.
- Generalised seborrhoea oleosa (Fig. 10.1).
- Waxy debris accumulates in the face folds and ears (Fig. 10.2).
- Malodorous.

Differential diagnosis

- Causes of secondary seborrhoea:
  - Ectoparasites, e.g. fleas, Cheyletiella.
  - Endocrine, e.g. hypothyroidism.
  - Dermatophytosis.
  - Thymoma.
  - Seborrhoeic dermatitis (Malassezia).

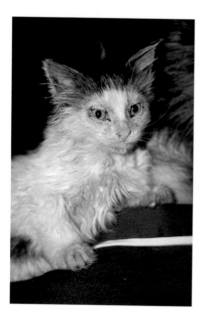

Fig. 10.1 Generalised primary seborrhoea in a young kitten.

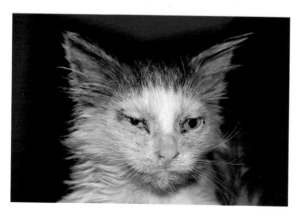

Fig. 10.2 Close up facial area Fig. 10.1.

Diagnosis

- History – especially in a young cat.
- Diagnostic rule-outs including:
  - Skin scrapings.
  - Acetate tape impression smears.
  - Fungal culture.
  - Endocrine function tests.
- Biopsy.
  - Secondary infection may be present.
  - Histopathology consistent with keratinisation defect.

Treatment

- Long term control required.
- Symptomatic treatment should consist of:
  - Topical therapy with antiseborrhoeic shampoos
  - Essential fatty acids.
  - Retinoids.
  - Steroids.

Topical therapy with antiseborrhoeic shampoos

- Many cats will tolerate regular shampoo therapy if they are started at a young age.
- Coat should be kept well groomed; clipping often helps.
- Shampoo is used once or twice weekly initially, then as required for maintenance.
- Shampoos suitable for:
  - Dry seborrhoea – sulphur, salicylic acid (Kerect, C Vet; Sebomild, Virbac).
  - Dry seborrhoea with secondary infection:
    Bacteria – ethyl lactate (Dermacleanse, C Vet; Etiderm, Virbac), chlorhexidine, sulphur, salicylic acid (Duoderma, C Vet).
    Bacteria/yeast – chlorhexidine, miconazole (Malaseb, Leo Labs).
  - Greasy seborrhoea – selenium sulphide (Seleen, Sanofi).
    N.B. Tar shampoos should not be used in cats.
  - Greasy seborrhoea with secondary infection – benzoyl peroxide (Paxcutol, Virbac).
- Shampoos for greasy seborrhoea are rarely needed for long term maintenance.
- Cats can be switched to dry seborrhoea shampoo, or potent degreasing shampoos can be alternated with milder products.
- After bath rinses containing essential fatty acids, moisturisers and humectants can be useful, e.g. Humilac, Virbac.

Essential fatty acids

- Omega-3, omega-6 fatty acid supplements successful in some cases.

Retinoids

- May be successful but there is no published data on their use in primary seborrhoea.

Steroids

- Used as a last resort when other problems are controlled.
- Prednisolone – 1.0 mg/kg to reduce greasiness, the lowest possible dose used on an alternate day basis for maintenance.

Ichthyosis (fish scale disease)

Cause and pathogenesis

- Very rare disease.
- Possibly equivalent to lamellar ichthyosis in man due to epidermal hyperproliferation.

Clinical signs

- Generalised grey scales, skin roughened.
- Malodorous seborrhoeic skin.
- Hyperkeratosis of foot pads and nasal planum.

Differential diagnosis

- In young kittens few other diseases present in this way.

Diagnosis

- Clinical signs.
- Skin biopsy.

Treatment

- Incurable disease needs aggressive long-term management.
- Symptomatic treatment as greasy primary seborrhoea.

Aplasia cutis

Cause and pathogenesis

- An inherited discontinuity of squamous epithelium.
- Mode of inheritance in the cat unknown.

Clinical signs

- Present at birth.
- Ulceration of the skin due to loss of epithelium.
- Any site, may be small deficits or extensive areas.

Differential diagnosis

- Trauma.
- Burns – mechanical, heat or chemical.

Diagnosis

- Clinical signs in a young kitten.
- Skin biopsy – complete absence of epidermis, hair follicles and glands.

Treatment

- Primary closure or skin grafting may repair small areas.
- Extensive areas – secondary infection common leading to death.

Eyelid coloboma

Cause and pathogenesis

- Congenital discontinuity of eyelid (Fig. 10.3).
- Breed incidence – Siamese.

Clinical signs

- Present at birth.
- Tends to be bilateral, usually upper eyelids.
- Lateral component of lid affected.

Differential diagnosis

- Trauma.
- Burns – mechanical, heat or chemical.

Diagnosis

- Clinical signs in a young kitten.

Treatment

- Primary closure or skin grafting may repair small areas.

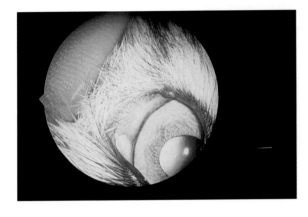

Fig. 10.3 Eyelid coloboma
(picture courtesy of P. Boydell).

Epidermolysis bullosa (EB)

Cause and pathogenesis

- Hereditary mechanobullous disease.
- Three subtypes have been identified:
  - ○ EB simplex – clefting occurs at the intraepidermal level.
  - ○ Junctional EB – clefting occurs at the intralamina lucida level.*
  - ○ Dystrophic EB – clefting occurs sublamina level.*

Clinical signs

- Present at birth or soon afterwards.
- Vesicles, bullae, ulcers, ulceration. Seen at mucocutaneous junctions, especially in the mouth and on paws (Fig. 10.4).
- Paronychia; claws often slough (Fig. 10.5).
- Defects in tooth enamel and retarded growth can also be seen.

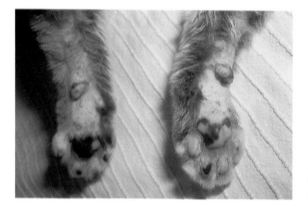

Fig. 10.4 Ulceration on paws with epidermolysis bullosa (picture courtesy of H. O'Dair).

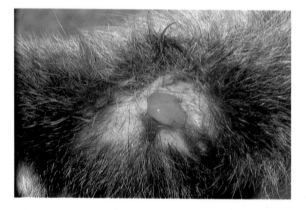

Fig. 10.5 Nail bed involvement in epidermolysis bullosa (picture courtesy of H. O'Dair).

---

* Identified in cats.

Differential diagnosis

- Other differential unlikely in view of the age of onset and clinical appearance.
- Trauma.
- Burns – mechanical, heat or chemical.

Diagnosis

- Clinical signs – present at birth or soon afterwards.
- Skin biopsy – dermal–epidermal separation.
- Electron microscopy and immunohistochemistry are required to determine the level of the cleavage and therefore the subtype of the disease.

Treatment

- None.
- Environmental management to minimise trauma to skin.
- Guarded prognosis.

DISORDERS OF HAIR AND HAIR GROWTH

- see Chapter 9

DISORDERS OF PIGMENTATION

Chediak–Higashi syndrome

Cause and pathogenesis

- Inherited autosomal recessive disease seen in blue Persian cats.
- Cats have giant lysosomes in the cells of numerous tissues including neutrophils and macrophages.
- Abnormal neutrophils exhibit delayed intracellular killing, leading to increased susceptibility to infection.

Clinical signs

- Young kittens.
- Breed incidence – blue smoke, yellow eyed Persian cats.
- Cutaneous signs:
  - Dilute coat colour – blue smoke.
  - Increased risk of bacterial and fungal infection (especially dermatophytic pseudomycetoma).
- Ocular signs:

- ○ Partial ocular albinism compared to normal copper coloured iris of blue Persian.
- ○ Photophobia.
- ○ Reduced fundic pigmentation red compared to normal yellow/green.
- ○ Congenital cataracts.
- Haematological signs:
  - ○ Abnormal platelet function leading to increased bleeding tendency.

Differential diagnosis

- Little else present with this range of clinical signs in this breed and colour of cat.

Diagnosis

- History and clinical signs.
- Trichography – hairs contain multiple large irregular clumps of melanin (macromelanosomes).
- Blood smear.
  - ○ Neutrophils and macrophages contain large eosinophilic granules (giant lysosomes).
  - ○ Platelet counts – normal (thrombocytopathy rather than thrombocyto-paenia).

Treatment

- Nothing available.
- Animals should be removed from any breeding programme.

DISORDER OF COLLAGEN FORMATION

Ehlers–Danlos (cutaneous asthenia, dermatosparaxis)

Cause and pathogenesis

- Inherited congenital defect in collagen formation.
- Tensile strength of skin reduced 10-fold – skin will tear easily.
- Dominant or recessive mode of inheritance.

Clinical signs

- Breed incidence – domestic short haired, long haired and Himalayan cats.
- Young kittens.
- Cutaneous signs:
  - ○ Skin soft, hyperextensible (Fig. 10.6), usually thin.
  - ○ Often hangs loosely in folds especially legs and throat.
  - ○ Tears easily to produce large gaping wounds.
  - ○ Heals quickly leaving 'cigarette paper' scars.

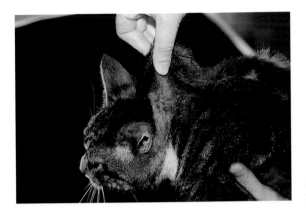

Fig. 10.6 Hyperextensible skin in cat with Ehlers–Danlos.

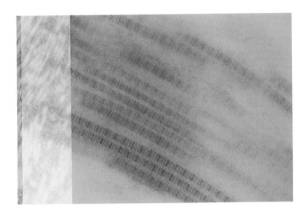

Fig. 10.7 Electron microscopy of well ordered collagen bundles from a normal cat.

- Non-cutaneous signs:
  - Joint laxity.
  - Ocular changes, e.g. lens luxations, cataract.

Differential diagnosis

- Hyperadrenocorticism.
- Feline acquired skin fragility.

Diagnosis

- Clinical signs – very characteristic.
- Extensibility index of dorsolumbar skin $= \dfrac{\text{vertical height of skin fold}}{\text{body length}} \times 100.$
- Extensibility index of affected cat greater than 19.0%.
- Skin biopsy can appear normal – in some cases dermis may be thinned and collagen bundles may be abnormal; special collagen stains may be useful.
- Electron microscopy – diagnostic (Figs 10.7 and 10.8).

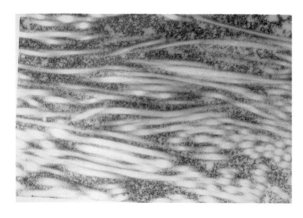

Fig. 10.8 Electron microscopy of disorganised abnormal collagen bundles from cat in Fig. 10.6.

Treatment

- Prevent animals from breeding.
- Environmental modification to reduce trauma to the skin.
- Vitamin C therapy of possible benefit – 50 mg per cat daily.

Chapter 11

Diseases Causing Abnormal Pigmentation

INCREASES IN PIGMENT

- Hyperpigmentation – increased pigment in skin or hair.
- Melanoderma – excessive pigment in skin.
- Melanotrichia – excessive pigment in hairs.

GENETIC CAUSES OF HYPERPIGMENTATION

Lentigo simplex

- Asymptomatic macular melanosis of young cats.

Cause and pathogenesis
- Unknown.

Clinical signs
- Breed incidence – domestic short haired and long haired orange cats.
- Age incidence – cats less than 1 year of age.
- Lesions found commonly on the lips, also nose (Fig. 11.1), gingiva and eyelids.
- Small uniformly black macules (1–9 mm in diameter) that enlarge and proliferate with time.
- Asymptomatic, non-pruritic, do not ulcerate.
- Do not undergo neoplastic transformation.

Differential diagnosis
- Pigmented neoplasms, e.g. melanoma, basal cell tumour.

Treatment
- None necessary – this is a cosmetic defect.

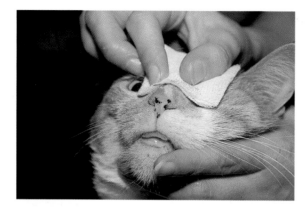

Fig. 11.1 Macular melanosis of planum nasale in an orange cat.

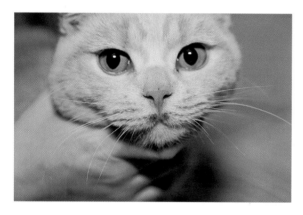

Fig. 11.2 Post inflammatory hyperpigmentation on nose.

ACQUIRED CAUSES OF HYPERPIGMENTATION

Post inflammatory hyperpigmentation

- Cats uncommonly produce post inflammatory hyperpigmentation.
- Can been seen secondary to:
  - ○ Infection – bacterial/fungal.
  - ○ Chronic pruritus secondary to allergy (Fig. 11.2) or ectoparasites.
  - ○ Endocrine imbalance.

Tumour hypermelanosis

- Many different tumours can appear as pigmented lesions including:
  - ○ Melanocytoma/melanoma.
  - ○ Basal cell tumour.
  - ○ Mastocytosis (urticaria pigmentosa).

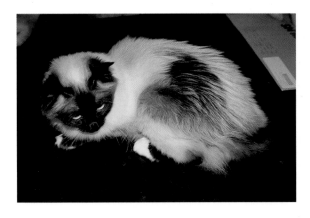

Fig. 11.3 Dark hair regrowth on the flanks after successful therapy of flank alopecia due to atopy.

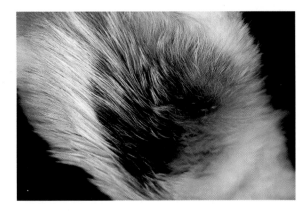

Fig. 11.4 Close up of hair in Fig. 11.3.

Feline acromelanism

- Naturally occurring coloration of the extremities is seen in particular breeds.
  ○ Siamese, Burmese, Himalayan and Balinese.
- A temperature dependent enzyme involved in melanin synthesis controls the colour.
- High environmental temperatures produce light hair, low temperatures dark hair.
- Physiological factors such as inflammation and alopecia can also influence colour.
- Many of these cats will regrow dark hair over an area that has been clipped for surgery or as hair is regrown after an inflammatory process (Figs 11.3 and 11.4).
- Hair will return to its normal colour after the next hair cycle.

DECREASES IN PIGMENTATION

- Hypopigmentation – decreased pigment in skin or hair coat.
- Leukoderma – lack of pigment in skin.
- Leukotrichia – lack of pigment in hair.

GENETIC CAUSES OF HYPOPIGMENTATION

Chediak–Higashi syndrome

- See Chapter 10.

Vitiligo

Cause and pathogenesis

- Rare autoimmune reaction thought to selectively destroy epidermal melanocytes.

Clinical signs

- Breed incidence – Siamese cats.
- Females may be predisposed.
- Young adults.
- Progressive macular depigmentation of nose, lips, eyelids, footpads, pinna, oral mucosa, scrotum and perianal areas.
- Diffuse generalised leukotrichia.
- Cat systemically well.
- Depigmentation may be temporary or permanent.
- Progressive repigmentation can occur after several years.

Differential diagnosis

- Systemic/discoid lupus erythematosus.
- Epitheliotrophic lymphoma.

Diagnosis

- Clinical signs.
- Skin biopsy – lack of melanocytes in lesional skin without inflammatory or degenerative changes.

Treatment

- Unsuccessful.

Waardenburg–Klein syndrome

Cause and pathogenesis

- Failure of in the migration and/or differentiation of melanoblasts.
- Autosomal dominant mode of inheritance with incomplete penetrance.

Clinical signs

- Cutaneous lesions.
- Complete lack of pigment in the hair and skin (white cats).
- Other lesions.
- Deafness.
- Heterochromia of irides.

Diagnosis

- Clinical signs.
- Skin biopsy – lack of melanocytes.

Treatment

- None.
- Animal should not be used for breeding.

ACQUIRED CAUSES OF HYPOPIGMENTATION

Post inflammatory hypopigmentation

- Hypopigmentation will occur secondary to any agent that destroys melanocytes or inhibits their ability to produce pigment.
- Causes include:
  - Trauma.
  - Burns – chemical, heat, cold (especially cryosurgery, irradiation).
  - Infection – fungal, bacterial.
  - Drugs – especially glucocorticoids.
  - Nutritional deficiencies – especially copper.
  - Neoplasia – epitheliotrophic lymphoma, squamous cell carcinoma.
  - Immune mediated disease, e.g. lupus erythematosus, pemphigus foliaceus (Fig. 11.5).

Idiopathic periocular leukotrichia

Cause and pathogenesis

- Precise cause is unknown.
- Precipitating factors include:

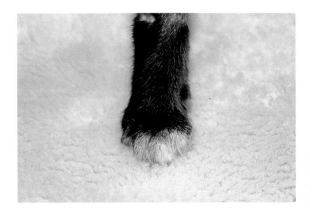

Fig. 11.5 Post inflammatory hypopigmentation of pedal hair after successful therapy for pemphigus foliaceus.

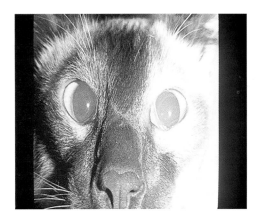

Fig. 11.6 Idiopathic periocular leukotrichia in a Siamese cat (picture courtesy of P. Boydell).

- ○ Oestrous.
- ○ Pregnancy.
- ○ Dietary deficiency.
- ○ Systemic illness (upper respiratory tract disease).

Clinical signs

- Breed predisposition – Siamese cats.
- Most commonly in females.
- Patchy or complete loss of hair pigment around both eyes (Fig. 11.6).

Differential diagnosis

- Post inflammatory hypopigmentation.
- Vitiligo.
- Aguirre syndrome.
- Systemic/discoid lupus erythematosus.

Diagnosis

- History and clinical signs.
- Skin biopsy as a diagnostic rule-out.

Treatment

- Therapy of any underlying disease.
- Hair will repigment within two hair cycles.

Aguirre syndrome

Cause and pathogenesis

- Unknown.

Clinical signs

- Breed predisposition – Siamese cats.
- Cutaneous lesions.
  - ○ Unilateral periocular depigmentation.
- Non-cutaneous lesions:
  - ○ Horner's syndrome.
  - ○ Corneal necrosis.
  - ○ Upper respiratory tract infections.

Differential diagnosis

- As idiopathic periocular leukotrichia.

Diagnosis

- Clinical signs in a predisposed breed.

Treatment

- Symptomatic.

Chapter 12

Keratinisation Disorders

Seborrhoea

- This is defined as abnormal formation of the cornified layer of the skin leading to scaling, and abnormal sebum production.
  - Seborrhoea oleosa describes greasy seborrhoea.
  - Seborrhoea sicca described dry seborrhoea.
- Neither term is a diagnosis but a description of a clinical finding.

Primary seborrhoea

- A rare disease covered in Chapter 10.
- This is a diagnosis of exclusion.

Secondary seborrhoea

- Almost any skin disease can produce seborrhoea.
- However, scaling can be mild in many cats due to their fastidious grooming behaviour, which removes much of the scale.
- Commonly seen with:
  - Endocrine disease – especially hyperthyroidism (Fig. 12.1), hyperadrenocorticism.
  - Nutritional factors – inappropriate diet, malabsorption, maldigestion syndromes.
  - Environmental factors, e.g. central heating, harsh topical therapy (insecticidal sprays, shampoos).
  - Inflammation – due to infection with dermatophytes, *Malassezia*, ectoparasites (Fig. 12.2).
  - Neoplasia – lymphoma.
  - Systemic disease – FeLV, FIV, FIP.
  - Inability to groom – dental disease, hypervitaminosis A.

Clinical signs

- Abnormal scaliness of coat.
- Coat is excessively dry or greasy.
- Ceruminous otitis externa common.

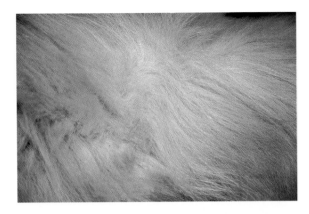

Fig. 12.1 Generalised seborrhoea oleosa in a hyperthyroid cat.

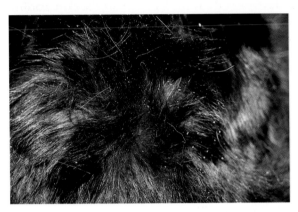

Fig. 12.2 Dorsal seborrhoea secondary to flea allergy.

- Precise signs and distribution depends on underlying diseases and cat's grooming activities.
- If an Elizabethan collar is used it will give a much truer indication of the distribution of scale.

Diagnosis

- History and clinical signs.
- Identification of underlying disease.
  - ○ Skin scrapings, hair pluckings, fungal culture.
  - ○ Endocrine function tests.
  - ○ Skin biopsy – often non-specific.

Treatment

- Correction of underlying disease where possible will allow natural resolution of the seborrhoea (1–2 months).
- Treatment of secondary infections, ectoparasites.
- Symptomatic therapy with shampoos or essential fatty acid supplementation may be useful (see primary seborrhoea in Chapter 10).

- Cats need to be continually reassessed but skin condition will change as primary disease is controlled.

Feline acne

- Uncommon keratinisation disorder.

Cause and pathogenesis

- Idiopathic condition caused by abnormal follicular keratinisation.
- Contributory factors may include:
  - Poor grooming habits.
  - Abnormal sebum production.
  - Primary keratinisation defects.
  - Stress associated with illness, especially viral effects.
  - Immunosuppression.
- Hormonal factors are not thought to be important.

Clinical signs

- No breed, sex or age predisposition.
- Lesions can occur as a single episode, appear cyclical or be constant.
- Early lesions
  - Comedones on chin and lips (often asymptomatic) (Fig. 12.3).
  - Papules and pustules develop later.
  - Pruritus mild.
- Chronic severe cases.
  - Secondary infection leads to folliculitis/furunculosis/cellulitis.
  - Pathogens include *Pasteurella multocida*, β-haemolytic streptococcus, *Staphylococcus*.
  - Oedema.

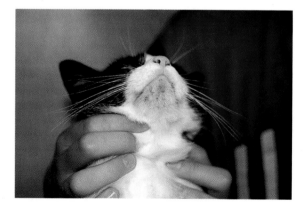

Fig. 12.3 Comedones on chin with feline acne.

   ○ Moderate–severe pruritus can lead to self-inflicted trauma and residual scarring.

Differential diagnosis

- Sebaceous adenitis.
- Eosinophilic granuloma complex.
- Dermatophytosis.
- Demodicosis.
- Allergy (food, atopy).
- *Malassezia*.

Diagnosis

- Clinical signs.
- Diagnostic rule out by skin scrapings, fungal culture, cytology.
- Skin biopsy – comedone formation, often with secondary infection.
- Culture and sensitivity may be useful to identify secondary infection.

Treatment

- Asymptomatic cases are essentially a cosmetic problem and can be left untreated.

Topical therapy

- Antiseborrhoeic shampoos:
  - ○ Mild degreasing products include those containing sulphur, salicylic acid (Kerect, C Vet; Sebomild, Virbac).
  - ○ Where additional antibacterial/yeast action is required ethyl lactate (Dermacleanse, C Vet; Etiderm, Virbac), chlorhexidine, sulphur, salicylic acid (Duoderma, C Vet), chlorhexidine, miconazole (Malaseb, Leo Labs).
  - ○ Potent degreasing products may be irritant to some cats. Benzoyl peroxide (Paxcutol, Virbac) has excellent degreasing and follicular flushing activity where tolerated.
- Antibacterial creams/lotions containing clindamycin, mupirocin, fucidin may also be useful where secondary infection is present.
- Topical vitamin A acid (Retin-A 0.05% cream) often useful, but irritancy can occur.

Systemic therapy

- Antibiotics based on culture and sensitivity where possible.
- Essential fatty acid supplementation may be useful.
- Steroids rarely indicated but may be given as a short course in sterile cases – 1–2 mg/kg daily by mouth.
- Retinoid therapy can be given in severe cases – Isotretinoin 1 mg/kg daily by mouth for up to 1 month, then every other day. These drugs are potent

teratogens and should be dispensed with care, especially to female owners of child-bearing age. Monitoring of the feline patient should include routine haematology, biochemistry especially liver function, triglycerides and cholesterol.

Feline tail gland hyperplasia

Cause and pathogenesis

- The tail gland in the cat is located along a dorsal line on the tail; it is rich in sebaceous and apocrine glands.
- Hyperplasia of the gland leads to the accumulation of waxy secretion on the surface of the skin.
- Commonly seen in entire males as 'stud tail' but hormonal link is unclear as can be seen in neutered cats and females.

Clinical signs

- No breed or age predilection; males may be over-represented.
- More commonly seen in catteries/cats that are confined.
- Excessive greasy secretions with scale and crust seen along dorsum of tail (Figs 12.4, 12.5).
- Overlying hair coat may be thinned.
- Skin may become hyperpigmented.
- Secondary infection is a rare complication.

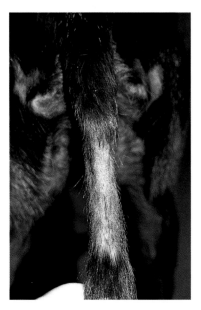

Fig. 12.4 Greasy seborrhoea on dorsum of tail 'stud tail'.

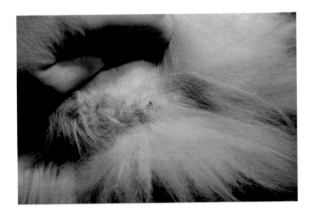

Fig. 12.5 Secondary infection on tail in a breeding tom cat with 'stud tail'.

Differential diagnosis

- Little else presents at this site with this clinical appearance.

Diagnosis

- Clinical signs.
- Bacteriological culture, tape strippings where secondary infection is present.

Treatment

- Castration of little benefit in entire males.
- Environmental changes to allow cat more freedom.
- Topical therapy – as feline acne.

Chapter 13

Psychogenic Dermatoses

- Psychogenic skin disease is over-diagnosed in the cat. True psychogenic disease is rare.
- Anxiety is usually the underlying psychogenic trigger and can induced by a variety of factors including:
  - Introduction of a new pet, relative, baby to the house.
  - House move.
  - Boarding in cattery.
  - Enforced confinement due to illness, especially orthopaedic problems.
  - Death of a companion human or another pet.
  - 'Bullying' by a dominant cat/dog in external environment.
- Overgrooming, where a chronic skin disease or local area of pain/abnormal sensation is left undiagnosed/untreated, can lead onto obsessive–compulsive behavioural patterns and self-inflicted trauma (see specific conditions).

Acral lick dermatitis (lick granuloma)

- A rare skin disease in the cat caused by over grooming.

Cause and pathogenesis

- Often both a psychogenic and an organic cause can be identified for the problem.
- Boredom or enforced confinement often concentrates cat's attention on one area.
- Underlying diseases include:
  - Fungal – kerion, pseudomycetoma.
  - Ectoparasites – fleas (Fig. 13.1).
  - Trauma – e.g. nerve damage causing abnormal sensation.
  - Allergy – atopy, food.
  - Neoplasia – mast cell tumour.
  - Orthopaedic problems, e.g. joint disease.
- All of these diseases as a minimum should be ruled out/treated before behaviour-modifying drugs are used.
- Traumatisation of the lesion establishes an itch/lick cycle leading to an obsessive–compulsive disorder (OCD).

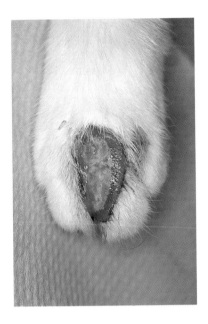

Fig. 13.1 Lick granuloma on foot of flea allergic cat (picture courtesy of D. Crossley).

Clinical signs

- No age, sex or breed predisposition.
- Lesions – single, unilateral, chronically thickened plaque or plaques or nodules, often with ulcerated surface.
- Usually seen cranial carpus or metacarpal area.

Diagnosis

- History and clinical signs.
- Laboratory rule-outs for underlying disease should always include:
  - Skin scrapings.
  - Hair plucking.
  - Impression smear.
  - Fungal/bacterial culture.
  - Fine needle aspirate plus biopsy if abnormal cell types are present.

Treatment

- Therapy of any underlying disease.
- Environmental modification to reduce stress, decrease boredom.
- Psychological drug treatment.
  - Anxiolytics.
    Phenobarbitone – 2.2–6.6 mg/kg orally twice daily.
    Diazepam – 1–2 mg/cat orally once or twice daily.
  - Tricyclic antidepressants.
    Amitriptyline – 0.5–1 mg/kg orally two or three times daily.

Fluoxetine – 1 mg/kg orally once daily.
Clomipramine (Clomicalm, Novactis) – 0.5–1 mg/kg orally once daily.
- ○ Endorphin blocker.
Naloxone – 1.0 mg/kg by subcutaneous injection as a single dose.
- Lesional treatment – should never replace a proper work-up.
  - ○ Physical prevention of licking – Elizabethan collar.
  - ○ Bandages are of little benefit in cats.
- Topical treatment – no benefit, as encourages overgrooming.
- Surgical removal – short-term remission – lesion often reproduced at same site.

Tail sucking

- Cats that suck their tails.

Cause and pathogenesis

- Usually associated with boredom or enforced confinement.
- May also be seen related to/exacerbated by systemic disease (Fig. 13.2).

Clinical signs

- Predisposed breed – Siamese.
- Distal 2–3 cm of the tail is wet due to sucking.
- No clinical lesions are present.

Differential diagnosis

- Conditions causing pruritus or pain to the tail or localised pain may be present in isolation or trigger psychological disease.
  - ○ Allergy.
  - ○ Parasites.
  - ○ Traumatic injury to tail base.
  - ○ Urolithiasis.

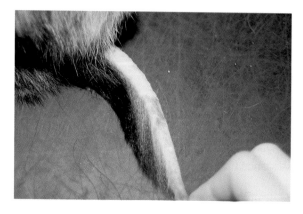

Fig. 13.2 Tail licking in a cat with chronic diarrhoea.

Diagnosis

- Clinical signs.
- Rule-outs of other conditions.

Treatment

- Anxiolytics or tricyclic antidepressants – dosage as acral lick dermatitis.

Foot licking

Cause and pathogenesis

- Rarely a psychogenic problem.
- Usually associated with paronychial problems.
- Underlying causes include:
  ○ Infection – bacteria, yeast.
  ○ Allergy – atopy/food (Fig. 13.3).
  ○ Autoimmune disease – pemphigus foliaceus.

Clinical signs

- Wetness of the feet due to licking often with associated hair loss.
- No primary lesions, no exudate from nail beds.

Differential diagnosis

- Medical causes of paronchyia and pododermatitis.

Treatment

- Treatment of underlying causes.
- Anxiolytic drug or tricyclic antidepressants – dosage as acral lick dermatitis.

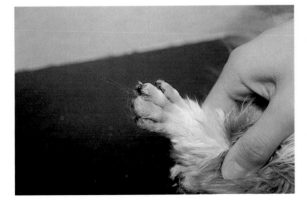

Fig. 13.3 Foot licking secondary to atopy.

Psychogenic dermatitis (neurodermatitis)

Cause and pathogenesis

- Anxiety is the most common trigger for true psychogenic dermatitis.
- Stress may lead to increases in adrenocorticotrophin hormone and melanocyte-stimulating hormone causing increased endorphin production.
- Endorphins are thought to protect the animal from stressful situations, although their production may reinforce the overgrooming activity.
- Obsessive grooming may be an extension of overgrooming induced by primary skin disease.

Clinical signs

- Breed predisposition – oriental breeds especially Siamese.
- In mild cases alopecia is the only finding, often with no associated inflammation.
- In severe cases alopecia is accompanied by marked self-inflicted trauma in the form of ulceration, often with the formation of eosinophilic plaques and secondary infection.
- Distribution patterns of alopecia can include:
  - Ventral alopecia.
  - Bilateral flank alopecia (Fig. 13.4).
  - Medial forelegs.
- Chronic lesions become lichenified and hyperpigmented.

Differential diagnosis

- Causes of traumatic alopecia.
  - Ectoparasites (fleas, *Cheyletiella*, *Otodectes*, lice, *Demodex*).
  - Allergy (atopy, food).
  - Dermatophytosis.
  - Seborrhoeic dermatitis (*Malassezia*).

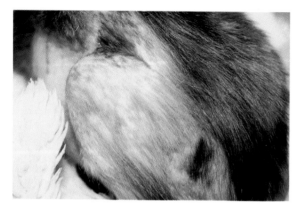

Fig. 13.4 Cat diagnosed as psychogenic alopecia after skin biopsy subsequently responded to improved ectoparasite control.

- Causes of non-pruritic alopecia.
  - Hypothyroidism (very rare).
  - Hyperadrenocorticism (very rare).
  - Telogen defluxion.
  - Anagen defluxion.
  - Acquired symmetrical alopecia.

Diagnosis

- These cases require an extensive work-up to rule out both traumatic and non-pruritic causes of alopecia.
- Investigations should include:
  - Skin scrapings.
  - Fungal cultures.
  - Allergy work-up including exclusion diets, intradermal testing.
  - Blood count – if there is an eosinophilia present then the condition is not psychogenic.
  - Skin biopsy of non-lesional areas often reveals normal skin.
  - Ectoparasite therapy.
  - Endocrine function tests.

Treatment

- Therapy of any underlying diseases.
- Psychological drug therapy – as acral lick dermatitis.

Chapter 14

Environmental Skin Diseases

Solar dermatitis

- Phototoxic reaction seen in poorly pigmented skin.

Cause and pathogenesis

- White skin, light skin or damaged skin that is not protected by sufficient hair is most susceptible.
- Primary solar dermatitis
  - Skin lesions are induced by sunlight in normal skin.
- Secondary solar dermatitis
  - Damaged e.g. scarred or depigmented, skin is further damaged by sunlight.
- Damage occurs during warm summer months by direct or reflected UVB sunlight.
- Highest risk periods are from 11.00 a.m. to 2.00 p.m.
- Pathogenesis is poorly understood, but reaction is phototoxic and thought to produce free radicals.

Clinical signs

- Blue-eyed white cats highly predisposed.
- Lesions seen on any sparsely haired and poorly pigmented skin (Fig. 14.1).
- Ear tips most common site, also margins of lower eyelids, nose and lips.
- Initial lesions – erythema and scale with alopecia usually asymptomatic.
- Chronic lesions – exudation, crusting, ulceration, painful often resulting in self-inflicted trauma.
- Age of onset is dependent on climate but can start at 3 months of age.
- Lesions become progressively worse each year.
- Neoplastic transformation can occur to squamous cell carcinoma.

Differential diagnosis

- Vasculitis.
- Discoid lupus erythematosus.
- Pemphigus foliaceus/erythematosus.
- Drug eruption.
- Dermatophytosis.

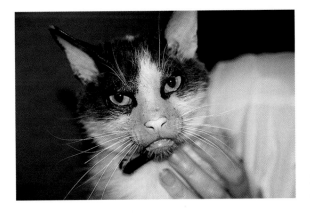

Fig. 14.1 Solar dermatitis affecting the nose.

- Neoplasia.
- Frostbite
- Cold agglutinin $\Big\}$ if presented during the winter.

Diagnosis

- History – sun exposure.
- Clinical signs – lesions found on predisposed areas.
- Skin biopsy – 'sunburn cells' or dyskeratotic keratinocytes.

Treatment

- Avoid further sun exposure especially between 9.00 a.m. and 3.00 p.m.
- Medical treatment.
- Photoprotection.
    - Sunblock – waterproof preparation – protection factor greater than 15.
- Systemic therapy.
    - Beta carotene and canthaxanthin can be given orally at a dose of 25 mg of active carotenoid.
    - Retinoids – etretinate 10 mg per cat orally may be useful.
- Surgical treatment.
    - Cosmetic amputation of the ears may be necessary, especially if there is possibility of early squamous cell carcinoma.

Actinic keratosis

Cause and pathogenesis

- Excessive exposure to ultraviolet light leads to solar damage to the skin.
- Especially seen in white cats that sunbathe.
- Premalignant lesions capable of becoming invasive squamous cell carcinoma.

Clinical signs

- Variable, can range from:
    - Single or multiple areas of erythema, hyperkeratosis and crusting to
    - Indurated crusted hyperkeratotic plaques (Fig. 14.2).
- Size 0.3–5.0 cm in diameter.
- Appear in lightly haired, and lightly pigmented skin.
- Predisposed sites include ear tips, nose, eyelids.

Differential diagnosis

- Neoplasia – especially squamous cell carcinoma, haemangiosarcoma.
- Pemphigus erythematosus/foliaceus.
- Systemic/discoid lupus erythematosus.
- Vasculitis.

Diagnosis

- History – especially white cat that sunbathes.
- Biopsy – atypia and dysplasia of epidermis.

Treatment

- Further sun avoidance imperative to avoid malignant transformation.
- Short term use of topical steroids.
- Surgical removal of affected area in severe cases.

Burns

- Burn management is often intensive and specialised.
- Only a brief outline of clinical signs and treatment will be provided here. The reader is referred to a more detailed text for further information.

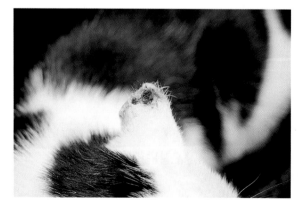

Fig. 14.2 Actinic keratosis of ear tips.

Cause and pathogenesis

- Types and extent of lesions depend on initial insult.
- Inciting factors:
  - Strong chemicals.
  - Electricity.
  - Solar radiation.
  - Microwave radiation.
  - Heat.
- Categories of burns.
  - Partial thickness burns involving epidermis/superficial dermis. Heal without scarring.
  - Full thickness burns – all cutaneous structures damaged. Extensive scarring without surgical treatment.

Clinical signs

Cutaneous lesions

- Often lesions not obvious for 24–48 hours but area very painful.
- Lesions dependent to some extent on type of burn.
- Skin hard and dry, hair may hide full extent of lesions.
- Secondary infection with Gram-negative organisms especially *Pseudomonas aeruginosa* occurs after 3–5 days leading to suppuration, often malodorous.

Non-cutaneous lesions

- These seen when greater than 25% of body involved.
- Septicaemia, shock, renal failure, anaemia.

Differential diagnosis

- Drug eruption.
- Pemphigus complex.

Diagnosis

- History.
- Clinical signs – tapering areas of coagulation necrosis of epidermis – with thermal or chemical burns.

Treatment

- In severe cases – general assessment is essential, especially of renal function, hydrated status.
- Skin lesions
  - Clean with antiseptic agent.
  - Debride.

○ Topical antibacterials, e.g. silver sulphadiazine, mupirocin.
○ Glucocorticoids contraindicated.

Frostbite

Cause and pathogenesis

- Caused through prolonged exposure to low environmental temperature or contact with frozen objects.
- Precise lesions depends on insult to skin.

Clinical signs

- Extremities affected – especially ear and tail tips, digits.
- Skin pale and cold whilst frozen; once thawed erythema, pain, necrosis and sloughing in severe cases.

Differential diagnosis

- Vasculitis – especially cold agglutinin disease.

Diagnosis

- History.
- Clinical signs.

Treatment

- Avoidance of cold.
- Rapid but gentle thawing of frozen tissue with warm water.
- Lesions will heal spontaneously.
- Surgical resection of necrotic tissue may be necessary.

Irritant contact dermatitis

Cause and pathogenesis

- This should be distinguished from contact hypersensitivity.
- Particularly common where cats have fallen into a chemical, e.g. paints, disinfectants (Fig. 14.3).
- Because cats are fastidious groomers they often ingest large amounts of toxic or corrosive material in attempts to clean their coats.
- Ingestion of the irritant may not only cause gastrointestinal ulceration but also signs of systemic poisoning.
- Types of irritant include:.
  ○ Corrosive – strong acid or alkaline causes immediate damage, severe reaction as a chemical burn.

○ Soaps, detergents, topical insecticides (especially flea collars, Fig. 14.4) – prolonged or repeated exposure is required.

Clinical signs

- Irritation occurs on hairless or sparsely haired skin.
- Shampoos, solvents, etc., can penetrate the hair coat and will cause more generalised signs where the chemical touches the skin.
- Lesions – papules and erythema, severe pruritus leading to self-inflicted trauma.
- Systemic signs depend on chemical.

Differential diagnosis

- Where the irritant is a liquid, it is usually still present in the coat and there are few other likely causes.
- Where the irritant is non-liquid and affects hairless areas.
  ○ Intradermal penetration by parasites, e.g. hookworm, *Strongyloides*.
  ○ Allergy (contact, atopy, food).

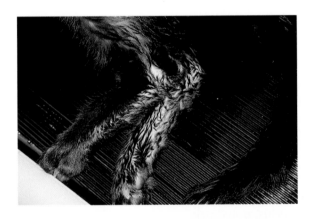

Fig. 14.3 Oil on legs of cat after falling into a drum of oil.

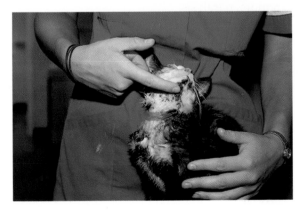

Fig. 14.4 Severe contact irritation after application of flea collar.

Diagnosis

- History – multiple animals affected if it is an environmental irritant.
- Clinical signs.
- Skin biopsy – non-diagnostic except as a rule-out.
- Provocative testing should be avoided especially if there is potential for severe reactions.

Treatment

- Identification of irritant substances plus removal.
- Symptomatic relief – short term steroids.
  - ○ Systemic prednisolone – 1 mg/kg once daily for 7–10 days.
  - ○ Topical steroid creams – short term use.

Thallium poisoning

Source

- Rodenticide now withdrawn from the market.

Clinical signs

- Acute toxicity – fatal within 4 days.
- Chronic toxicity – cutaneous lesions appear within 2 days of ingestion.
- Cutaneous signs:
  - ○ Erythema and alopecia of periocular skin, mucocutaneous junctions, feet, perineum and ventrum.
  - ○ Footpads hyperkeratotic and ulcerated.
  - ○ Lesions can become more generalised with time.
- Systemic signs:
  - ○ Mild early signs – gastroenteritis, polydipsia.
  - ○ Nervousness, convulsions, tremors, paralysis.

Differential diagnosis

- Drug eruptions.
- Necrolytic migratory erythema.
- Systemic lupus erythematosus.
- Erythema multiforme.

Diagnosis

- History and clinical signs.
- Skin biopsy – degenerative changes in hair follicle and surface epithelium.
- Detection of thallium in the urine.

Treatment

- Supportive care with fluids, antibiotics and B complex vitamins.
- Activated charcoal or Prussian blue (250 mg/kg by mouth in divided doses) may trap thallium in the bowel to allow its excretion in faeces.

Traumatic injury

Cause and pathogenesis

- A very common cause of skin lesions in cats.
- Inciting causes include:
  - Bite wounds (see also Chapter 2).
  - Road traffic accidents.
  - Gun shot/air pellet wounds.

Clinical signs

- Entirely dependent on the underlying cause.
- Bite wounds.
  - Made by cats – usually form a single puncture wound that heals to form an abscess.
  - Made by dogs – often no puncture wound but massive external bruising and internal injury (Fig. 14.5).
- Road traffic injuries.
  - Often superficial excoriation of the skin.
  - Hair may be singed.
  - Coat may be oil stained.
  - Often damage to the nails.
  - Deglooving injuries commonly seen on the extremities (Fig. 14.6).
- Gunshot wounds
  - Often localised pain and only a small entry wound (Fig. 14.7).
  - Hole often contains inverted hair.

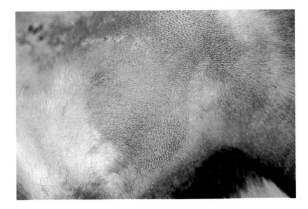

Fig. 14.5 Bruising to flanks caused by dog bite.

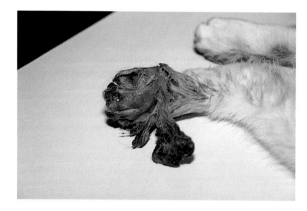

Fig. 14.6 Deglooving injury on hind leg following a road traffic accident.

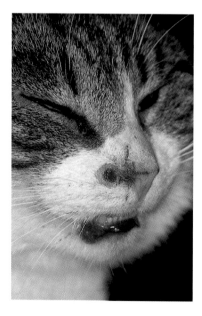

Fig. 14.7 Air gun pellet entry wound on face (picture courtesy of D. Crossley).

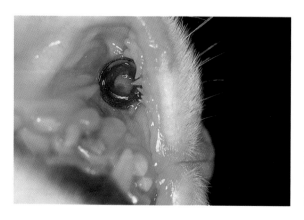

Fig. 14.8 Air gun pellet from cat in Fig. 14.7 located inside the mouth (picture courtesy of D. Crossley).

○ Identification of the pellet can rarely be made by visual inspection (Fig. 14.8).

Diagnosis

- History and clinical signs.
- Radiography in two planes may be useful in cases of gunshot wounds.

Treatment

- Symptomatic – dependent on presenting signs.

Chapter 15

Nutritional Skin Diseases

Nutritional requirements of cats

- Cats have very precise dietary requirements and skin disease can occur through inadequate/unbalanced nutrition.
- Cats have a protein requirement of 25–30%, which is much higher than that of dogs (18–20%). Kittens require 35% protein in their diet.
- Cats require taurine in their diets – deficiency leads to retinal degeneration and blindness.
- Cats cannot convert the fatty acid linoleic acid to arachidonic acid. Cats must therefore consume preformed arachidonic acid which is found in animal tissue.
- Cats cannot convert β-carotene in plants to vitamin A. They must therefore consume preformed vitamin A which is found in animal tissue.
- Cats cannot convert the amino acid tryptophan to the B vitamin, niacin. Cats have a high requirement for niacin in their diets.
- Cats also have a high requirement for vitamin B-6 (pyridoxine).

Formulation of special diets for cats

- Indications.
  - Investigation of food intolerance/allergy.
  - Investigation of immune mediated disease/drug eruption.
- Types of diet:
  - Home cooked – these usually contain a single protein source and occasionally a carbohydrate. Such a 'pure' diet will not contain colourants, additives, etc., but is nutritionally incomplete and will lead to deficiencies if fed for prolonged periods.
  - Proprietary tinned or dried prescription diets. Not as pure as the home cooked alternative, but balanced and unlikely to cause any signs of dietary deficiency. Such diets should be considered when the cat to be food-trialled is immature and still growing.

Protein deficiency

Cause and pathogenesis

- Normal hair growth requires 25–30% of the animal's total daily protein intake.
- Feeding low protein diets.

- ○ Feeding kittens/cats on dog food which has inadequate protein.
- ○ Low protein prescription diets fed inappropriately for renal/hepatic disease.
- Systemic illness – numerous causes of protein loss, including protein-losing nephropathy, gastroenteropathy, hepatopathy, chronic blood loss.

Clinical signs

- Cutaneous signs will often precede weight loss.
- Generalised scaling.
- Loss of hair pigment.
- Poor hair growth, hair thinner, dry, brittle (Fig. 15.1).
- Patchy alopecia.

Diagnosis

- History and clinical signs.
- Investigation of dietary deficiency or search for source of protein loss.

Treatment

- Poor quality diets – improve protein levels in diet.
- Systemic illness.
  - ○ Correction of underlying diseases.
  - ○ Specific dietary supplementation with the use of prescription diets.

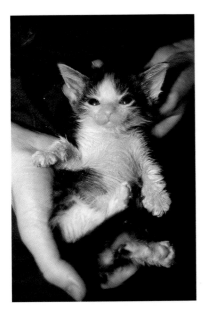

Fig. 15.1 Generalised hair loss and seborrhoea oleosa in a protein deficient kitten.

Fatty acid deficiency

Cause and pathogenesis

- Essential fatty acids should constitute at least 2% of the caloric intake of the diet.
- Cats require both linoleic acid and arachidonic acid; both are omega-6 fatty acids.
- Rare disease caused through:
  - Inadequate diet – especially poorly formulated or preserved foods, seen particularly in young kittens, cats fed a vegetarian diet.
  - Internal disease.
    Gastrointestinal disease – inflammatory or neoplastic lesions leading to malabsorption/maldigestion.
    Chronic renal or hepatic disease.

Clinical signs

- Cutaneous signs:
  - Generalised scaling, loss of lustre of hair coat.
  - Chronic changes – seborrhoea oleosa plus ceruminous otitis.
  - Secondary infection with bacteria or yeast common.
  - 'Hot spots' – areas of acute moist dermatitis.
  - Non-allergic miliary dermatitis.
  - Impaired wound healing.
- Other signs.
  - Abnormal reproductive function.

Differential diagnosis

- Primary seborrhoea.
- Other causes of secondary seborrhoea.

Diagnosis

- History and clinical signs.
- Laboratory rule-outs of causes of secondary seborrhoea.
- Skin biopsy – orthokeratotic hyperkeratosis with no underlying epidermal hyperplasia.
- Routine haematology, biochemistry, FeLV, FIP, FIV.

Treatment

- Where the problem is caused by an inadequate diet then feeding a balanced diet is preferable to fatty acid supplementation.
- Identification of underlying disease.
- In cases where there is a chronic disease, balanced supplements containing omega-6 fatty acids should be given. If these are unavailable:

○ Natural sources of linoleic acid include soya or corn oil.
○ Natural sources of arachidonic acid include poultry fat or lard.

Pansteatitis

Cause and pathogenesis

- Rare disease caused by an excessive consumption of unsaturated fatty acids with inadequate dietary intake of antioxidants.
- Diets are usually high in oily fish – especially tuna, sardines.
- The accumulation of reactive peroxides (end products of rancidification) in adipose tissue produces yellow discoloration of body fat. So called 'yellow fat disease'.

Clinical signs

- Predisposing factors – young and obese cats.
- Generalised signs:
  ○ Depression, febrile.
  ○ Inability to jump up or move freely.
  ○ Anorexia.
  ○ Ascites uncommon but raises suspicion of FIP as a major differential diagnosis.
- Cutaneous signs:
  ○ Cutaneous pain when handled due to inflammation of subcutaneous fat. Usually generalised inflammation of all fat deposits.
  ○ Nodular subcutaneous deposits of fat or fibrous tissue, especially in the groin and on the ventral abdomen (Fig. 15.2).
  ○ Overlying skin usually appears normal unless traumatised by the cat.

Differential diagnosis

- Infectious causes of nodular skin disease include:
  ○ Bacterial infections such as:

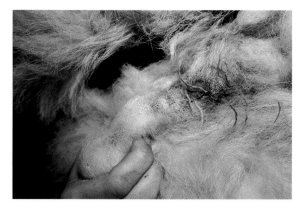

Fig. 15.2 Pansteatitis affecting the groin.

        Bacterial pseudomycetoma.
        Mycobacteria.
        Yersinia pestis (plague).
        Actinomycosis.
        Actinobacillosis.
        Nocardiosis.
  - Dermatophytic pseudomycetoma.
  - Fungal mycetoma.
- Sterile causes of nodular skin disease:
  - Neoplasia.
  - Foreign body.

Diagnosis

- History of high fat diet.
- Clinical signs.
- Skin biopsy – fat is characteristically brown/yellow/orange when samples are taken.
  - Special stains to rule out infectious causes.
  - Lobular/septal panniculitis with or without fat necrosis and mineralisation.

Treatment

- Dietary changes to feed a balanced cat food. Appetite stimulants and/or force feeding may be needed to encourage the cat to eat the new diet.
  - Cyproheptadine – 2 mg twice daily by mouth or
  - Diazepam – 1 mg twice daily by mouth can both be used as appetite stimulants.
- Vitamin E supplementation (alpha tocopherol) – 20–50 mg/kg body weight by mouth once daily. Should be given for one month beyond clinical cure.
- Glucocorticoids as a short course at anti-inflammatory doses:
  - Prednisolone – 1–2 mg/kg once daily by mouth for 7 days then every other day for 10 days.

VITAMIN RELATED DERMATOSES

Vitamin A deficiency

Cause and pathogenesis

- Rare disease caused through inadequate levels of vitamin A in the diet.
- Seen in animals fed a vegetarian diet. Cats cannot convert β-carotene in plants to vitamin A and need preformed vitamin A from meat.
- Vitamin A is required for normal skin formation and ocular function.

Clinical signs

- Generalised signs:
  - ○ Retinal degeneration, photophobia.
  - ○ Weakness of hind legs.
  - ○ Reproductive failure.
- Cutaneous signs:
  - ○ Poor coat, alopecia, generalised scale.

Diagnosis

- History – especially related to a poor or inappropriate diet.
- Clinical signs.
- Skin biopsy – follicular hyperkeratosis.

Treatment

- Provision of a balanced diet containing meat.
- Vitamin A supplementation often not necessary.
- Toxicity can occur through excess supplementation.

Hypervitaminosis A

Cause and pathogenesis

- Seen in cats that are fed a diet rich in vitamin A.
- This may be due to over supplementation, especially with cod-liver oil or diets containing large quantities of liver.

Clinical signs

- Cumulative disease – cats tend to be elderly (>8 years of age).
- Generalised signs:
  - ○ Anorexia, weight loss.
  - ○ Periarticular exostoses – especially forelimb and neck, leading to stiffness and eventual cervical spondylitis.
- Cutaneous signs:
  - ○ Hyperaesthesia.
  - ○ Cat reluctant to groom, leading to poor quality unkempt coat and generalised seborrhoea (Fig. 15.3).

Differential diagnosis

- Cutaneous lesions:
  - ○ Seborrhoea related to chronic systemic disease.
  - ○ Hyperthyroidism.

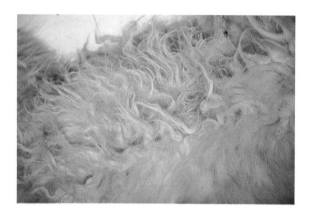

Fig. 15.3 Unkempt coat in a cat with hypervitaminosis A. Cat is unable to groom due to cervical spondylitis.

Diagnosis

- History and clinical signs.
- Radiographic signs of bony changes.

Treatment

- Institution of a balanced diet.
  - ○ This can be difficult, as cats can become obsessive about liver-based food.
  - ○ Force feeding and appetite stimulants may be necessary (see treatment of pansteotitis).
- Prognosis very guarded – often changes are irreversible.

Vitamin B deficiencies

- Rare disease caused through deficiency of biotin, riboflavin, niacin.

Causes

Biotin deficiency

- Diets high in uncooked eggs.
- Chronic antibiotic therapy.

Riboflavin deficiency

- Diets without meat or dairy products, particularly seen in cats put on a vegetarian diet.

Niacin deficiency

- Diets low in protein/high in corn.

Clinical signs

Biotin deficiency

- Periocular alopecia plus crusting on face, neck, body.
- Non-allergic miliary dermatitis.
- Lethargy, diarrhoea.

Riboflavin deficiency

- Periocular and ventral seborrhoea.
- Cheilosis.

Niacin deficiency

- Pellagra – dermatitis, neuritis, glossitis.
- Ulceration of mucous membranes.

Treatment of vitamin B deficiencies

- Balanced commercial cat foods.
- Brewer's yeast.
- B complex injection.

Chapter 16

Miscellaneous Skin Diseases

Feline plasma cell pododermatitis

- Rare skin disease affecting the footpads of cats.

Cause and pathogenesis

- Precise cause unknown.
- Clinical findings include tissue plasmacytosis, hypergammaglobulinaemia.
- These findings plus cat's response to immune modulating drugs suggest an immune mediated cause.
- Some cases show a seasonal pattern.

Clinical signs

- No breed, sex or age predilection.
- Cutaneous signs:
  - Early/mild signs:
    Soft painless swellings of multiple footpads on multiple paws (Fig. 16.1).
    Central metatarsal or metacarpal pads usually affected.
    Surface of pads often appear purple with white cross hatching.
    Pads feel soft/mushy.
  - Severe signs:
    Cat is lame, footpads very painful.
    Pads may become ulcerated, often burst open (Fig. 16.2).
    Secondary infection common.
- Other signs:
  - Plasma cell stomatitis.
  - Immune mediated glomerulonephritis.
  - Renal amyloidosis.

Differential diagnosis

- Infectious causes of pyogranulomatous disease include:
  - Bacterial infections such as:
    Bacterial pseudomycetoma.
    Mycobacteria.
    Actinomycosis.

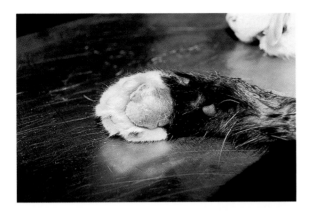

Fig. 16.1 Plasma cell pododermatitis showing purple cross-hatching of pad.

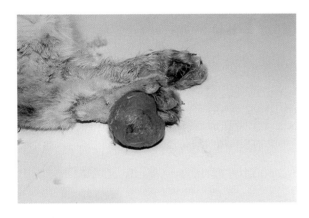

Fig. 16.2 Severe case of plasma cell pododermatitis after the pad has split.

    Actinobacillosis.
    Nocardiosis.
- Dermatophytic pseudomycetoma.
- Fungal mycetoma.
- Viral disease.
    Calicivirus.
    Herpesvirus.
    Poxvirus.
- Sterile causes of nodular skin disease:
  - Neoplasia.
  - Foreign body.
- These all usually only affect a single footpad.

Diagnosis

- History and clinical signs.
- Fine needle aspirates reveals numerous plasma cells with small numbers of lymphocytes and neutrophils.

- Biopsy – perivascular dermatitis with heavy plasma cell infiltrate.
- Cultures usually negative.
- Blood samples:
  - Hypergammaglobulinaemia.
  - ANA, FeLV, FIV occasionally positive but inconsistent findings.

Treatment

- Benign neglect in non-painful cases as regression can occur spontaneously.
- Medical treatment can be used with:
  - Prednisolone – 2.2 mg/kg twice daily by mouth. Tapering down to lowest possible alternate day levels once clinical remission has occurred.
    Usually takes about 2–3 weeks to see benefits.
    Maximal improvement is seen in 10–14 days.
  - Chrysotherapy. Gold injection (Solganol, Schering) – initially as an intramuscular test dose of 1 mg, then at a dose of 1 mg/kg weekly until remission obtained.
    Lag period for gold is 6–12 weeks; other drugs (e.g. steroids) may have to be maintained during this time.
    After remission the gold is given every 2 weeks.
    Monitoring.
    Induction period – full blood count and urine analysis weekly.
    Long term – monthly blood and urine checks.
- Surgical treatment
  - In severe cases that are unresponsive to therapy, badly affected footpads may have to be amputated.

Lichenoid dermatoses

Cause and pathogenesis

- Unknown – possible immune mediated disease.
- Can be seen as a response to ectoparasites.

Clinical signs

- No age, breed or sex predilection.
- Asymptomatic, flat topped papules with scaly surface.
- Can occur in groups or can coalesce to form plaques.
- Any site on the body.
- No systemic signs associated with lesions.

Differential diagnosis

- Dermatophytosis.
- Sterile granulomatous disease.

- Neoplasia.
- Eosinophilic granuloma complex.

Diagnosis

- Clinical signs.
- Laboratory rule-outs of other disease, including fungal culture and skin scrapings.
- Skin biopsy – lichenoid and hydropic interface dermatitis.

Treatment

- Treatment of underlying cause if established.
- Excellent prognosis – a benign disease.
- Often with benign neglect these lesions will self-resolve in 6 months to 2 years.

Idiopathic sterile granuloma and pyogranulomas

Cause and pathogenesis

- Unknown – these sterile lesions are thought to be immune mediated.
- Underlying flea hypersensitivity has been identified in some cases.

Clinical signs

- Two syndromes are recognised:
  - ○ Preauricular plaques.
    No breed predilection, older males may be predisposed.
    Papules coalesce to form orange-yellow well-circumscribed plaques.
    Pruritus moderate–severe.
    Palpation of lesions leads to red/purple discoloration.
  - ○ Papulonodular lesions.
    No breed predilections, young females may be predisposed.
    Pruritic papules and nodules on the head and pinnae (Fig. 16.3).
    Lesions erythematous to violaceous.

Differential diagnosis

- Infectious granulomas (bacterial, fungal).
- Foreign body granulomas.
- Neoplasia.
- Eosinophilic granuloma.
- Granulomatous sebaceous adenitis.

Diagnosis

- Clinical signs.
- Tissue culture (fungal, aerobic and anaerobic bacteriological culture).

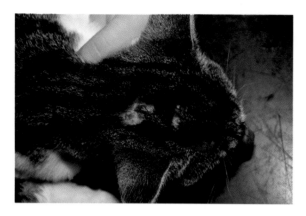

Fig. 16.3 Sterile papulonodular lesions on head.

- Skin biopsy.
    - Preauricular plaques – diffuse granulomatous dermatitis, narrow grenz zone containing multinucleate giant cells.
    - Papulonodular lesions – perifollicular pyogranulomatous dermatitis.

Treatment

- Solitary lesions – surgical excision.
- Multiple lesions – prednisolone – 2.0–4.0 mg/kg once daily by mouth until regression, usually 10–14 days.
- Many cats' lesions resolve spontaneously over 6–9 months without therapy.
- Remission can be long-lived.

Sebaceous adenitis

- Very rare idiopathic skin disease in the cat.

Cause and pathogenesis

- Precise aetiology unclear, possibly:
    - Developmental/inherited defects leading to sebaceous gland destruction.
    - Immune mediated attack against components of sebaceous gland.
    - Keratinisation disorder.
    - Abnormality of lipid metabolism.

Clinical signs

- Initial lesions found on head, pinnae and neck.
- Chronically, lesions will generalise.
- Multifocal annular areas of crust and scale.
- Hairs easily epilated.
- Prominent follicular casts on hairs.
- Alopecia.

Differential diagnosis

- Dermatophytosis.
- Hyperadrenocorticism.
- Demodicosis.
- Cutaneous neoplasia (lymphoma, thymoma).
- Seborrhoeic dermatitis (*Malassezia*).

Diagnosis

- Clinical signs.
- Laboratory rule-outs of other conditions, including skin scrapes and fungal cultures.
- Trichography – prominent follicular casts.
- Skin biopsy – granulomatous/pyogranulomatous sebaceous adenitis.
- Chronic lesions – sebaceous gland destroyed.

Treatment

- Response to treatment can be disappointing and often difficult to assess as sebaceous adenitis can be cyclical in nature.
- Topical treatment.
  - ○ Antiseborrhoeic shampoos containing salicylic acid, sulphur and ethyl lactate plus emollient rinses.
- Systemic treatment.
  - ○ Essential fatty acids – oral administration of products containing omega-6 and omega-3 fatty acids has been shown to be useful in some cases.
  - ○ Prednisolone – 1 mg/kg daily for 10 days, then alternate days, tapering to lowest possible dose.

Sterile panniculitis

Cause and pathogenesis

- Can occur as:
  - ○ Solitary lesions which can be associated with trauma, foreign bodies or be idiopathic.
  - ○ Multiple lesions associated with immune mediated disease such as systemic lupus erythematosus, pancreatic dysfunction, or idiopathic disease.

Clinical signs

- No age, sex or breed predilection.
- Solitary lesions.
  - ○ Deep seated cutaneous nodule often ulcerated with an oily discharge – yellow/haemorrhagic fluid.
  - ○ Common sites include ventral abdomen (Fig. 16.4) and ventrolateral thorax.

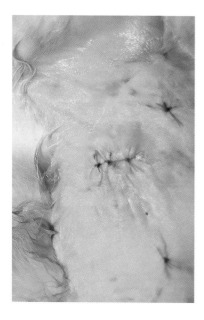

Fig. 16.4 Panniculitis on ventral abdominal skin; sutures indicate site of biopsy.

- Multiple lesions.
  - Cutaneous lesions – as solitary lesions but usually occur in crops on dorsum and flanks.
  - Non-cutaneous signs:
    Inappetence, depression, lethargy.
    Abdominal pain, vomiting – especially if there is pancreatic involvement.

Differential diagnosis

- Infectious panniculitis of bacterial, mycobacterial, actinomycotic, fungal origin.
- Sterile pyogranulomatous disease.
- Neoplasia.

Diagnosis

- Clinical signs.
- Cytology of direct smear and fine needle aspirate – neutrophils, foamy macrophages.
- Skin biopsy – excisional biopsy of a nodule if possible, special stains necessary to rule out infective organisms.
- Culture – sterile.
- Blood samples – antinuclear antibody, pancreatic function tests.

Treatment

- Solitary lesions – surgical excision.
- Multiple lesions.

- ○ Prednisolone – 4 mg/kg by mouth once daily for 3–8 weeks until clinical remission, then tapering off over 1 month. Some cases require long term alternate day therapy.
- ○ Vitamin E – 400 IU by mouth twice daily (given 2 hours before or after feeding).

Hypereosinophilic syndrome

- Rare disease manifesting with persistent idiopathic eosinophilia with diffuse infiltration of the skin and internal organs.

Cause and pathogenesis

- Unknown – may be an immune mediated disease.

Clinical signs

- No age, breed or sex predilection.
- Cutaneous lesion – uncommon.
  - ○ Maculopapular erythema, severe pruritus, and excoriation at any site.
- Systemic signs – common:
  - ○ Typically there is infiltration of bone marrow, lymph nodes, liver, spleen and gastrointestinal tract.
  - ○ Diarrhoea, vomiting and weight loss are common.

Differential diagnosis

- Cutaneous lesions:
  - ○ Eosinophilic granuloma complex.
  - ○ Idiopathic sterile granulomatous disease.
  - ○ Ectoparasitic infestation.
  - ○ Allergy (food, atopy).

Diagnosis

- History and clinical signs.
- Peripheral eosinophilia.
- Cytology of skin lesion – eosinophils and basophils.
- Skin biopsy – superficial and deep eosinophilic perivascular dermatitis.

Treatment

- Poor prognosis – the disease is poorly responsive to therapy and systemic disease is rapidly fatal.
- Where cutaneous lesions predominate, the prognosis is better and cats will survive 2–4 years. In these cases high doses of steroids may be beneficial.

Ulcerative dermatitis with linear subepidermal fibrosis

Cause and pathogenesis

- Unknown – trauma, injection reactions, infection and foreign bodies do not contribute.
- May be a form of vascular insult that leads to the production of a non-healing ulcer.

Clinical signs

- No sex, age or breed predilection.
- Lesions are solitary and occur over the dorsal neck and shoulder area (Fig. 16.5).
- Non-painful, pruritus variable.
- Non-healing ulcer initially 0.5–1.0 cm in diameter enlarges over several weeks.
- Thick adherent crusting over the surface with peripheral thickened skin.

Differential diagnosis

- Injection reaction.
- Trauma – especially bite wound.
- Panniculitis (infectious or sterile).
- Neoplasia – especially squamous cell carcinoma.
- Burn (cold, heat, chemical).

Diagnosis

- History and clinical signs.
- Carefully performed cultures are negative.
- Skin biopsy – linear subepidermal band of superficial fibrosis.

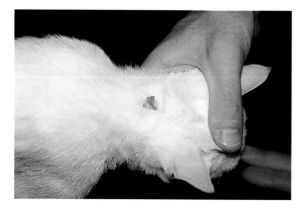

Fig. 16.5 Idiopathic ulcerative dermatitis affecting the back of the neck.

Treatment

- Wide surgical excision carries a good prognosis, recurrence uncommon.
- Glucocorticoid therapy may be useful in some cases.
  - Prednisolone – 4mg/kg daily by mouth in divided doses until clinical remission, then tapering to alternate day and withdrawal. If no response is seen within 4 weeks surgical excision should be undertaken.

Perforating dermatitis

Cause and pathogenesis

- Unknown – in man these conditions are often associated with internal malignancy, diabetes mellitus or chronic renal failure. No such association has been identified in the cat.
- Lesions thought to be caused by some abnormality in collagen metabolism.

Clinical signs

- Any site can be affected.
- Lesions consist of multiple firm conical hyperkeratotic yellow-brown masses.
- Appear often in clusters, forming lines.
- Non-pruritic, non-painful.
- Removed with difficulty.

Differential diagnosis

- Cutaneous horn.
- Dermatophytosis.

Diagnosis

- Clinical signs.
- Skin biopsy – exophytic mass containing keratin and degenerate collagen.

Treatment

- Ascorbic acid (vitamin C) – 100mg every 12 hours by mouth.
- Lesions resolve within 30 days.
- Long-term treatment is usually required.

Acquired skin fragility

- Rare disease characterised by thin fragile skin.

Cause and pathogenesis

- Multifactorial disease it can be associated with:
  - ○ Hyperadrenocorticism.
  - ○ Iatrogenic Cushing's syndrome.
  - ○ Diabetes mellitus.
  - ○ Hepatic and/or renal disease.
  - ○ Overuse of progestational compounds.
  - ○ Idiopathic.

Clinical signs

- No sex or breed predilection, although middle aged–old cats predisposed.
- Skin thin, easily torn by minor trauma.
- Large sheets of skin can be lost.
- Partial alopecia often present (Fig. 16.6).

Differential diagnosis

- Cutaneous asthenia.
- Hyperadrenocorticism.
- Iatrogenic Cushing's syndrome.
- Pancreatic paraneoplastic alopecia.

Diagnosis

- History – cutaneous asthenia is seen in very young cats present from birth.
- Clinical signs.
- Biochemistry – dynamic function tests to rule out endocrine disease.
- Skin biopsy – difficult in view of the fragility of the skin.
  - ○ Dermal collagen fibres thin and disorganised.

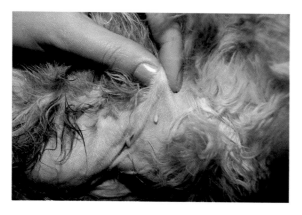

Fig. 16.6 Partial alopecia and thin inelastic skin in cat with acquired skin fragility.

Treatment

- Even if an underlying cause is identified skin changes appear to be irreversible.
- Surgical repair unsuccessful.
- Very poor prognosis.

Idiopathic facial dermatitis in Persians

- Uncommon pruritic facial disease seen in the Persian cat.

Cause and pathogenesis

- Unknown.
- Cats may have a sebaceous gland abnormality.
- A genetic basis of the disease may be possible.

Clinical signs

- Young Persian cats of either sex appear predisposed (<5 years).
- Lesions confined to the head and neck.
- Erythema, alopecia and marked self-inflicted trauma.
- Thick black exudation with crusting of hairs (Fig. 16.7).
- Ceruminous otitis seen in approximately 50% of cases.
- Secondary bacterial and yeast infection common.
- Herpetic eye disease may be present concurrently.

Differential diagnosis

- Allergy (atopy, food, fleas).
- Demodicosis.
- Dermatophytosis.
- Idiopathic sterile pyogranulomatous disease.

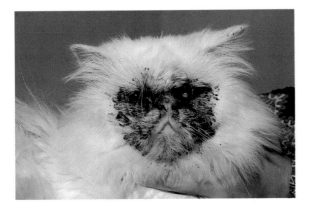

Fig. 16.7 Idiopathic facial dermatitis in a Persian.

Diagnosis

- History, clinical signs in a predisposed breed.
- Cultures for bacteria, yeast secondary problem.
- Other findings include negative FeLV, FIV assays, dermatophyte cultures.
- Occasional positive skin test reactivity.
- Skin biopsy – interface dermatitis, sebaceous hyperplasia.

Treatment

- Unrewarding, poor prognosis.
- Topical therapy with antiseborrhoeic shampoos is of limited short-term benefit.
- Limited response to systemic therapy with antibiotics, glucocorticoids, immune modulators, essential fatty acids.

Chapter 17

Eosinophilic Allergic Syndrome

- Eosinophilic allergic syndrome is not a specific disease entity but a spectrum of cutaneous reaction patterns exhibited by the cat to a wide variety of different disease processes.
- There can therefore be no one drug which can be used to control the clinical signs.
- Eosinophilic allergic syndrome encompasses both the eosinophilic granuloma complex and also miliary dermatitis, so that it can be subdivided into four categories:
  ○ Indolent ulcer (eosinophilic ulcer, rodent ulcer).
  ○ Eosinophilic plaque.
  ○ Allergic miliary dermatitis.
  ○ Eosinophilic granuloma (linear granuloma, collagenolytic granuloma).
- Miliary dermatitis has been included in the grouping as it is now widely accepted as being part of the same disease process. Histologically, lesions of miliary dermatitis can be indistinguishable from those of the eosinophilic plaques.
- Any of the different lesions of the complex can occur in the same cat concurrently.
- Each disease will be described for cause and pathogenesis, clinical signs, differential diagnosis and diagnosis. Investigation of all four diseases to determine the underlying cause is very similar and will be dealt with in a separate section at the end of the chapter, as will therapy.

Indolent ulcer

Cause and pathogenesis

- Cutaneous, mucocutaneous, or oral lesions. Many have underlying immune mediated aetiologies including allergies; other lesions may be a manifestation of excessive grooming leading to a purely mechanical trauma to the area.

Clinical signs

- No age, breed or sex predilection (females may be at higher risk).
- Usually found on the upper lip unilaterally (bilaterally less commonly; Fig. 17.1).

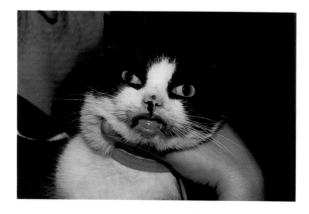

Fig. 17.1 Bilateral indolent ulcers affecting the top lips.

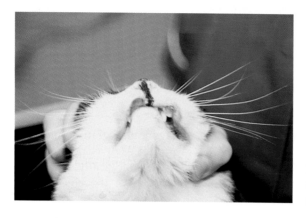

Fig. 17.2 Underside of lips of cat with indolent ulceration showing typical appearance.

- Other lesions found in oral cavity.
- Lesions are well circumscribed, red-brown in colour.
- Alopecic often ulcerated with a raised border (Fig. 17.2).
- Size 2 mm to 5 cm.
- Usually asymptomatic – rarely pruritic or painful.
- Peripheral lymphadenopathy common.

Differential diagnosis

- Infectious ulcers (bacterial, viral, fungal).
- Trauma.
- Neoplasia (squamous cell carcinoma, mast cell tumour).

Diagnosis

- This should initially be aimed at confirming the lesion as an indolent ulcer.
- Once this has been established, investigation should be as for all four diseases to identify an inciting cause (see later).
- Impression smears – stained with Diff Quik to assess degree of infection.

- Cultures – carefully performed samples are sterile.
- Haematology – unremarkable, eosinophilia rare.
- Biopsies useful only as a diagnostic rule-out.
  - ○ Selection of biopsy site – deep wedge or punch biopsy of margin of ulcer to include normal skin if possible.
  - ○ Findings – non-specific – superficial perivascular to interstitial dermatitis often with fibrosing dermatitis. Eosinophils an inconsistent finding.

Eosinophilic plaque

Cause and pathogenesis

- Common cutaneous reaction pattern seen in cats.
- Most cats have underlying allergic conditions.
- Overlap occurs between miliary dermatitis lesions and eosinophilic plaques: the former condition cannot be easily differentiated from the latter histologically.
- Miliary dermatitis probably represents a multifocal distribution of lesions, eosinophilic plaques the same disease process in a localised form.

Clinical signs

- No age or breed predilection although females may be predisposed.
- Most occur on the abdomen and medial thighs, although occasionally they can be identified at mucocutaneous junctions.
- Lesions may be single or multiple.
- Highly pruritic lesions.
- Raised round to oval well-demarcated erythematous lesions (Figs 17.3 and 17.4).
- Lesions often exudative and ulcerated.
- Lesions vary in size from 0.5 to 5.0 cm in diameter (Fig. 17.5).
- Regional lymphadenopathy common.

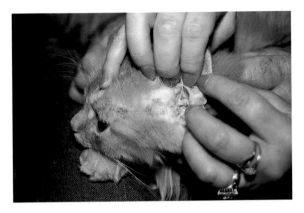

Fig. 17.3 Eosinophilic plaques on the face.

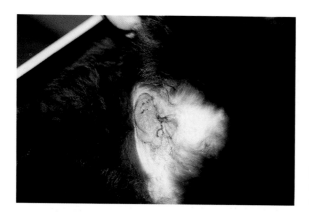

Fig. 17.4 Well demarcated eosinophilic plaque on the ventral abdomen.

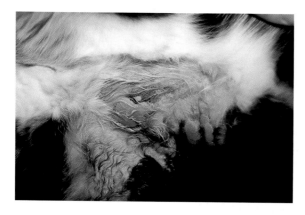

Fig. 17.5 Extensive area of eosinophilic plaque formation on ventral abdomen.

Differential diagnosis

- Infectious granulomas (bacterial, viral, fungal).
- Neoplasia (mast cell tumour, metastic mammary carcinoma, lymphoma).

Diagnosis

- To confirm the lesion as an eosinophilic plaque.
- Clinical appearance.
- Impression smears – stained with Diff Quik to assess degree of infection.
- Cultures – carefully performed samples are sterile.
- Haematology – eosinophilia a constant finding.
- Biopsies are diagnostic.
  - ○ Selection of biopsy site – erythematous plaques with minimal erosion or self-inflicted trauma.
  - ○ Findings – hyperplastic superficial and deep perivascular dermatitis with eosinophilia – interstitial or diffuse eosinophilic dermatitis.

Allergic miliary dermatitis

Cause and pathogenesis

- Miliary dermatitis is a multifactorial cutaneous reaction pattern. It can be divided into allergic and non-allergic causes.
- Most cases of miliary dermatitis are produced by cutaneous hypersensitivity reactions; these may be to environmental allergens, ectoparasites or drugs, so called allergic miliary dermatitis.
- Histopathologically there is overlap between this disease and eosinophilic plaques, which are thought to be a more localised form of the same disease.
- Non-allergic miliary dermatitis is considered under other headings (see dermatophytosis, pemphigus foliaceus, staphylococcal folliculitis, cowpox).

Clinical signs

- No breed, age or sex predilection has been identified.
- Multiple discrete erythematous papules with adherent brown-black crust (Fig. 17.6).
- The crusted papules represent primary lesions and are not the product of self-inflicted trauma.
- Lesions are typically found on dorsal lumbosacral area (Fig. 17.7), caudomedial thighs and neck.
- Pruritus moderate–severe.
- Chronic resolving lesions may appear as small melanotic macules.

Differential diagnosis

- Non-allergic causes of miliary lesions including:
  - Pemphigus foliaceus.
  - Dermatophytosis.
  - Staphylococcal folliculitis.
  - Dietary imbalances (biotin, fatty acid deficiency).
  - Feline poxvirus.

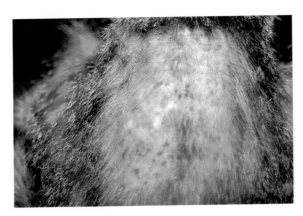

Fig. 17.6 Multiple discrete lesions of miliary dermatitis.

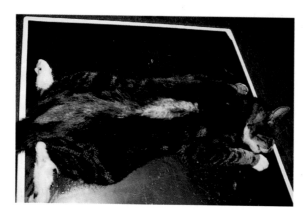

Fig. 17.7 Miliary dermatitis showing typical distribution along the dorsum.

Diagnosis

- To confirm the lesion as miliary dermatitis.
- Clinical appearance.
- Impression smears – stained with Diff Quik to assess degree of infection.
- Cultures – bacterial and fungal cultures carefully performed samples are sterile.
- Haematology – eosinophilia a consistent finding, often with basophilia.
- Biopsies are non-diagnostic but help as a diagnostic rule-out.
  - Selection of biopsy site – non-traumatised recently erupted papules, especially between the shoulder blades.
  - Findings – superficial and deep perivascular – interstitial dermatitis with eosinophilic infiltrate accompanied by mast cells.

Eosinophilic granuloma

Cause and pathogenesis

- A common cutaneous, mucocutaneous and oral mucosal lesion.
- Thought to be a manifestation of allergic disease.

Clinical signs

- No age or breed predilection, although females may be at higher risk.
- Lesions most commonly seen on caudal thighs (Fig. 17.8), face and oral cavity; however, can be seen at almost any site (Fig. 17.9).
- Appear as well circumscribed raised yellow-pink plaques with a linear configuration (Fig. 17.10).
- Ulcerated surface can be covered in pinpoint white foci of collagen degeneration.
- Peripheral lymphadenopathy variable.
- Pruritus usually mild.

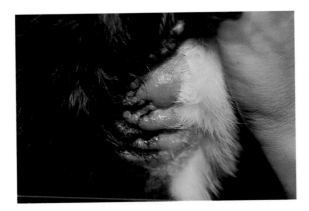

Fig. 17.8 Eosinophilic granuloma on the caudal thigh.

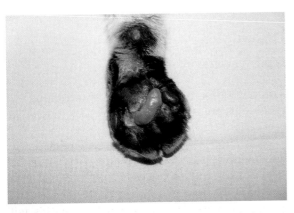

Fig. 17.9 Eosinophilic granuloma on the footpad.

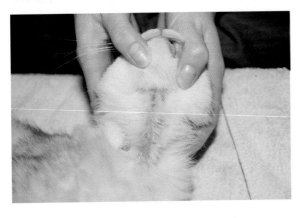

Fig. 17.10 Eosinophilic granuloma showing typical configuration on the neck.

- Chin oedema – asymptomatic swelling of the lower lip commonly caused by eosinophilic granuloma (Fig. 17.11).

Differential diagnosis

- Infectious granulomas (bacterial, viral, fungal).
- Neoplasia (mast cell tumour, metastic mammary carcinoma, lymphoma).

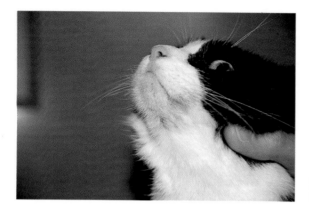

Fig. 17.11 Chin oedema caused by an eosinophilic granuloma.

Diagnosis

- To confirm the lesion as an eosinophilic granuloma.
- Clinical appearance.
- Impression smears – stained with Diff Quik to assess degree of infection.
- Cultures – carefully performed samples are sterile.
- Haematology – eosinophilia a consistent finding.
- Biopsies are diagnostic.
  - Selection of biopsy site – wedge biopsy from ulcerated area with white foci with minimal erosion or self-inflicted trauma to include a normal margin of skin.
  - Findings – nodular to diffuse granulomatous dermatitis with multifocal areas of collagen degeneration. Eosinophils and multinucleated giant cells are common.

Investigation of eosinophilic allergic syndrome

- Investigation should be undertaken when the cat is identified as having one or more of the following based on diagnostic tests to eliminate other differentials (such tests may include cytology, fungal culture, and skin biopsy):
  - Indolent ulcer.
  - Eosinophilic plaque.
  - Allergic miliary dermatitis.
  - Eosinophilic granuloma.
- The following protocol should be undertaken in all cases of eosinophilic allergic syndrome, but definitely in all cases that are:
  - Poorly responsive to anti-inflammatory therapy.
  - Recurrent.
  - Severe and/or multiple (i.e. more than one component of the syndrome is present).

Ectoparasite assessment

- Wet paper test for fleas.
- Acetate tape from coat for superficial parasites, e.g. *Cheyletiella, Otodectes, Trombicula*, lice, fur mites and flea faeces.
- Superficial skin scrapings for superficial parasites as above.
- Empirical therapy for ectoparasites should be undertaken even if no evidence is found on samples. The fastidious grooming habits of the cat can efficiently remove most parasites from the coat.
  - Adulticide therapy of cat plus all in-contact animals with, e.g. Fipronil spray (Frontline, Merial).
  - Environmental treatment insecticidal sprays:
    Permethrin/cyromazine (Staykil, Novartis).
    Pyrethrin/methoprene (Vet Kem Acclaim, Sanofi).

Food trial

- This can be started at the same time as the ectoparasite control or after 1 month's empirical therapy for parasites.
- Food should either be:
  - Home cooked to contain an unusual protein source not normally consumed by the cat, or
  - Proprietary selected protein hypoallergenic diet (for a more detailed discussion of such diets see section on food allergy in Chapter 7).
- Food trial should be for a minimum of 4–8 weeks.

Drug withdrawal

- Where any drugs have been prescribed before commencement of the lesions these should, where possible, be discontinued.

Allergy testing

- Where intradermal allergy testing is available it should be undertaken as the next diagnostic step.
- This allows identification of environmental allergens such as house dust mites, pollens, dust, animal danders and fungal moulds (for a more detailed discussion of such tests see section on atopy in Chapter 7).

Therapy

- This ideally should not be undertaken until the cat has had strict parasite control.
- However, it can be used in combination with parasite control when the cat is uncomfortable on initial presentation.
- Therapy should not replace even the most basic of work-ups.

- Inflammatory therapy can be started if the lesions are sterile, i.e. negative cultures and no bacteria on impression smears.

Medical therapy

- Anti-inflammatory therapy should not be given for more than 3–4 weeks at induction dose rates.
  - ○ Therapy should be reassessed if no clinical improvement is seen by this stage.
  - ○ Once lesions have resolved therapy should be tapered and withdrawn.
  - ○ Where atopy is identified long-term treatment is required, at lowest possible maintenance dose rates.
    Prednisolone – 4.4 mg/kg orally every 24 hours until lesions have resolved.
    Dexamethasone – 0.4 mg/kg orally every 24 hours until lesions have resolved.
    Triamcinolone – 0.8 mg/kg orally every 24 hours until lesions have resolved.
  - ○ Where the cat is difficult to medicate with tablets:
    Methylprednisolone acetate – 20 mg/cat subcutaneously for two injections 2 weeks apart.
- Where intradermal allergy testing identifies environmental allergens, specific avoidance therapy or desensitising vaccines can be used.
- Immunosuppressive therapy may be used in severe cases that are unresponsive to steroids (for details on monitoring see section on pemphigus in Chapter 7).
  - ○ Chlorambucil (Leukeran) – 0.1–0.2 mg/kg every 24–48 hours.
  - ○ Gold injection (Solganol, Schering) – initially as an intramuscular test dose of 1 mg, then at a dose of 1 mg/kg weekly until remission obtained.
    Lag period for gold is 6–12 weeks; other drugs (e.g. steroids) may have to be maintained during this time.
- Other drugs
  - ○ Progestational compounds such as megoestrol acetate, or medroxyprogesterone acetate are effective in many cases but the side effects of such drugs outweigh any therapeutic benefits and they should not therefore be used.
  - ○ Essential fatty acid supplementation with omega-3 and omega-6 fatty acid containing products has been shown to be useful in some cases of miliary dermatitis and eosinophilic granulomas.

Surgical therapy

- Other modes of therapy that have occasionally been successful include radiotherapy, cryotherapy, laser therapy and surgical excision.

Chapter 18

Neoplastic and Non-neoplastic Tumours

- This chapter is not designed to be a definitive guide to neoplasia in the cat. Only commonly occurring skin tumours will be described.
- The reader is referred to more specialised texts for further details.

EPITHELIAL NEOPLASIA

Cutaneous papilloma

- See viral diseases in Chapter 6.

Squamous cell carcinoma

- Common malignant neoplasm derived from keratinocytes.
- Locally invasive, slow to metastasise (except those arising from digits).
- Aetiology – sun damaged skin, chronically damaged skin and papilloma virus have all been implicated.

Age incidence

- Approximately 9 years.

Breed predisposition

- No breed or sex predilection.
- White cats (short-haired or long haired) have a 13-fold increased risk of developing squamous cell carcinoma due to their lack of skin and hair pigment.

Appearance

- Proliferative – papillomatous often ulcerated (Fig. 18.1).
- Ulcerative – crateriform crusted ulcers (Fig. 18.2).
- Lesions can have overlying cutaneous horn.

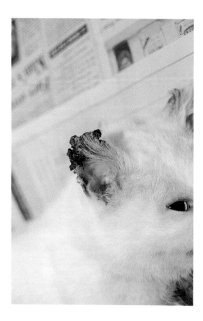

Fig. 18.1 Papillomatous proliferation on the ears due to squamous cell carcinoma.

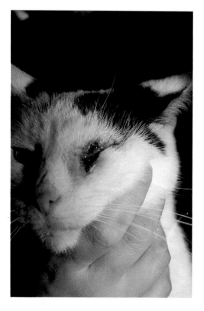

Fig. 18.2 Crusted ulceration caused by squamous cell carcinoma of eyelid.

- Site – head (80%) especially ear tips (54%) and eyelids (19%).
- Other sites can be affected but much less commonly.
- Lesions of clawbed invade bony tissue and metastasise more frequently.

Diagnosis

- Clinical signs.
- Biopsy – keratin cords, pearls.

Treatment

- Prognosis in the cat depends on the degree of differentiation of the tumour.
- 50% of cats with poorly differentiated tumours live only 12 weeks.
- Options.
  - Surgical excision offers a good prognosis for lesions of the pinnae and nose.
  - Cryosurgery also offers good prognosis for lesions around the head.
  - Electrosurgery.
  - Hyperthermia.
  - Radiotherapy.

Benign feline basal cell tumour

- Uncommon benign neoplasm derived from epithelial basal cells.
- Carries a good prognosis.

Age incidence

- 8–12 years.

Breed predisposition

- Himalayan and Persian cats.
- No sex predilection.

Appearance

- Solitary, occasionally multiple.
- Firm rounded well circumscribed lesions 1–2 cm in diameter.
- Often melanotic, usually ulcerated and alopecic.
- Site – head, neck limbs and dorsal trunk.

Diagnosis

- Clinical signs.
- Biopsy – well circumscribed symmetric proliferation of basaloid cells. Cells are arranged in tightly packed lobules.

Treatment

- Surgical excision.
- Electrosurgery.
- Cryosurgery.
- Benign neglect.

Basal cell carcinoma

- Common low-grade malignant neoplasm derived from small pluripotential cells within the basal cell layers of epidermis and adnexae.
- The incidence of recurrence and metastasis is very low.

Age incidence

- 7–10 years.

Breed predisposition

- Siamese cats.
- No sex predilection.

Appearance

- Usually solitary, well circumscribed, firm to cystic, 0.5–10 cm in diameter.
- Often melanotic, usually ulcerated and alopecic.
- Site – head, neck and thorax (Fig. 18.3), also eyelids and nasal planum.

Diagnosis

- Clinical signs.
- Biopsy – three different forms can be identified on histopathology:
  - Solid basal cell carcinoma – very common.
  - Keratinising basal cell carcinoma – rare in the cat.
  - Clear cell basal cell carcinoma – uncommon.

Treatment

- Surgical excision.
- Electrosurgery.
- Cryosurgery.
- Benign neglect.

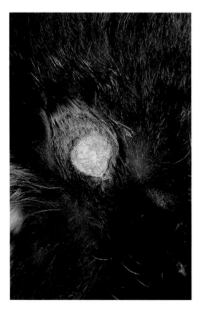

Fig. 18.3 Well demarcated basal cell carcinoma on thorax.

Trichoepithelioma

- Uncommon benign neoplasm of hair follicle.
- Rarely invasive or metastatic.

Age incidence

- Greater than 5 years.

Breed predisposition

- Persian cats.

Appearance

- Usually solitary but can be multiple, solid or cystic, well circumscribed, 0.5–15 cm in diameter.
- Commonly ulcerated and alopecic.
- Site – head, limbs and tail.

Diagnosis

- Biopsy.

Treatment

- Surgical excision.
- Cryosurgery.
- Electrosurgery.
- Benign neglect.

Pilomatrixoma

- Rare neoplasms derived from hair matrix cells.
- Rarely invasive or metastatic.

Age incidence

- Greater than 5 years.
- No sex predilection.

Breed predisposition

- Not described.

Appearance

- Well circumscribed solid and/or cystic tumour 1–10 cm in diameter.
- Site – shoulder, lateral thorax and dorsum.

Diagnosis

- Biopsy.

Treatment

- Surgical excision.
- Cryosurgery.
- Benign neglect.

Sebaceous gland tumour

- Uncommon neoplasms derived from sebocytes.
- Account for about 3% of all feline skin tumours.
- Rarely metastasise or recur.

Age incidence

- 10 years of age or older.
- No sex predilection.

Breed predisposition

- Persians.

Appearance

- Three different forms are recognised on histopathology:
  - ○ Sebaceous hyperplasia – very common in the cat. Elevated umbilicated lesion, 0.5 cm in size, usually multiple.
  - ○ Sebaceous adenoma – uncommon. Elevated lesion usually polyploid and ulcerated. Solitary mass >0.5 cm.
  - ○ Sebaceous carcinoma – rare. Solitary red intradermal nodule, alopecic, poorly circumscribed.

Diagnosis

- Biopsy important to differentiate the three forms.

Treatment

- Surgical excision important for carcinoma, which is locally invasive but rarely metastasises.
- Cryosurgery.
- Electrosurgery.
- Benign neglect in benign disease; not in the case of sebaceous carcinoma.

Sweat gland tumour

- Uncommon neoplasm derived from either glandular or ductal components of the apocrine sweat glands. May be benign or malignant.

Age incidence

- Greater than 10 years.
- No sex predilection.

Breed predisposition

- Apocrine sweat gland carcinomas may be more common in Siamese.

Appearance

- Solitary, well circumscribed, 0.3–3 cm in diameter.
- Occasionally ulcerated, may be cystic and often blue/purple in colour.
- Site – head (especially the cheek), pinna, neck, axilla, limbs and tail. Primary tumour can metastasize to paws.

Diagnosis

- Biopsy – different histological types are recognised. 80% are malignant.

Treatment

- Surgical excision.
- Cryosurgery.
- Electrosurgery.
- Benign neglect in non-malignant cases.

Ceruminous gland tumours

- Uncommon neoplasm derived from the modified apocrine glands of the external ear canal, the ceruminous glands.
- May be benign or malignant.
- Carcinomas are locally invasive and may metastasise to local lymph nodes.

Age incidence

- 6–13 years.
- No sex predilection.

Breed predisposition

- None.

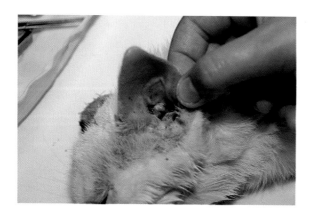

Fig. 18.4 Ceruminous gland adenoma in external ear canal.

Appearance

- Present with signs of chronic otitis externa.
- Chronic inflammation may predispose to neoplasia.
- Adenomas tend to be exophytic pedunculated masses with variable degrees of ulceration (Fig. 18.4).
- Carcinomas tend to be infiltrative, erosive and ulcerated.

Diagnosis

- Biopsy – approximately 55% of ceruminous gland tumours are malignant in the cat.

Treatment

- Surgical excision.
  - Pedunculated tumours can be easily removed.
  - Infiltrative tumours require lateral wall resection or total ear canal ablation.
- Radiation therapy may be necessary as an adjunct to surgery for carcinomas.

MESENCHYMAL TUMOURS

Mast cell tumour

- Common neoplasm derived from mast cells.
- May be cutaneous (see below) or visceral.
- Most tumours are benign and metastases are rare.

Age incidence

- Average age 10 years.
- Males predisposed.

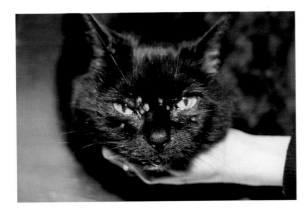

Fig. 18.5 Multiple mast cell tumours on the head.

Breed predisposition

- Siamese cats predisposed.

Appearance

- Very variable in appearance and size.
- Range from nodules and papules (Fig. 18.5) to alopecic masses and ulcerated plaques 0.2–5.0 cm in diameter.
- All tumours contain vasoactive substances that can produce localised oedema, inflammation and, rarely, anaphylactic shock if palpated.
- Site – head and neck.
- Systemic signs – gastro/duodenal ulceration and defective blood coagulation.

Diagnosis

- Cytology – impression smear, fine needle aspirate taken with care – mononuclear cells containing prominent granules.
- Biopsy – care is needed to differentiate mast cell tumours from other round cell tumours and eosinophilic plaques.
- Surgical staging of no benefit in the cat as it does not correlate with biological activity.

Treatment

- Single or multiple tumours.
- Surgical excision – where possible by wide excision 3 cm beyond palpable tumour.
- Medical treatment of no benefit.

Urticaria pigmentosa

- A benign proliferative mast cell disorder.

Age incidence

- Young cats <1 year of age.

Breed predisposition

- Described in Himalayans.

Appearance

- Macular erythema and hyperpigmentation around the mouth, chin, neck and eyes.

Diagnosis

- Biopsy – mast cell proliferation, epidermal hypermelanosis.

Treatment

- Non-spontaneous regression over a period of a few months.

Fibroma

- Uncommon benign neoplasm arising from fibroblasts.
- Non-invasive and non-metastatic.

Age incidence

- Older cats.
- No sex predilection.

Breed predisposition

- None.

Appearance

- Solitary, dome shaped pedunculated well-circumscribed nodules.
- Variable size.
- Site – limbs, flanks, groin.

Diagnosis

- Biopsy.

Treatment

- Surgical excision.
- Cryosurgery.
- Electrosurgery.
- Benign neglect.

Fibrosarcoma

- Common neoplasm derived from fibroblasts.
- Some are viral induced by feline sarcoma virus (FeSV). FeSV is a mutant of FeLV and therefore all FeSV positive cats are also FeLV positive.
- Solitary fibrosarcomas have also been associated with injection site reactions (especially FeLV and rabies).
- Rapidly growing, infiltrative metastasis <20%, usually to lungs.

Age incidence

- Any age.
- No sex predilection.
- Cats <5 years more prone to FeSV induced fibrosarcomas.
- Cats >5 years resistant to oncogenic effects of FeSV and thus do not produce tumours or else have benign spontaneously regressing lesions.

Breed predisposition

- Domestic shorthaired cats may be at increased risk.

Appearance

- Irregular and nodular, poorly circumscribed and firm.
- Variable size, often alopecic and ulcerated (Fig. 18.6).
- Single tumours usually seen in older cats (>5 years) and are not FeSV associated.

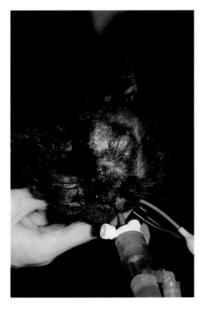

Fig. 18.6 Fibrosarcoma on face showing typical poorly circumscribed alopecic ulcerated appearance.

- Multicentric tumours seen in cats <5 years and are FeSV associated.
- Site – head, limbs, dorsum and abdomen.

Diagnosis

- Biopsy.

Treatment

- Wide surgical excision – recurrence rate after surgery high.
- Other therapy of limited benefit.

Haemangioma

- Rare benign neoplasm derived from endothelial cells of blood vessels.

Age incidence

- Older than 10 years, males predisposed.

Breed predisposition

- None.

Appearance

- Well circumscribed, round blue or red-black nodules 0.5–4.0 cm in diameter.
- Site – ears, face, neck and limbs.

Diagnosis

- Biopsy.

Treatment

- Surgical excision.
- Cryosurgery.
- Electrosurgery.
- Benign neglect.

Haemangiosarcoma

- Uncommon malignant neoplasm derived from endothelial cells of blood vessels.
- Solar damaged skin may be more susceptible, especially pinnae of white haired cats.
- Local recurrence very common.
- Rate of metastasis low.

Age incidence

- Greater than 10 years.
- Males predisposed.

Breed predisposition

- None.

Appearance

- Dermal haemangiosarcoma – solitary (especially if solar induced), poorly circumscribed red or dark blue plaques and nodules less than 2 cm in diameter.
- Subcutaneous haemangiosarcoma – poorly circumscribed dark red or blue black spongy masses up to 10 cm in diameter.
- Haemorrhage, alopecia and ulceration common with both forms (Fig. 18.7).
- Sites – head, pinnae, limbs, inguinal and axillary regions.

Diagnosis

- Biopsy.

Treatment

- Poor prognosis.
- Radical surgical excision – amputation if on limb.
- Chemotherapy – poor response.

Lipoma

- Uncommon benign neoplasms derived from subcutaneous lipocytes.

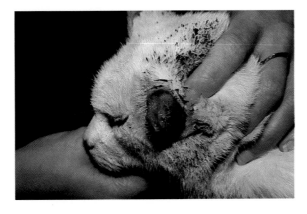

Fig. 18.7 Dermal haemangiosarcoma on ear of elderly cat.

Age incidence

- Greater than 8 years.
- No sex predilection.

Breed predisposition

- Siamese.

Appearance

- Usually single well circumscribed, soft fleshy dome-shaped tumours 1–30 cm in diameter.
- Site – over thorax, abdomen and proximal limbs.

Diagnosis

- Fine needle aspirate – cells stained for lipid.
- Biopsy.

Treatment

- Surgical excision – lesions can be reduced in size if animal loses weight.
- Benign neglect.

Liposarcoma

- Rare malignant neoplasms derived from subcutaneous lipoblasts.
- Locally infiltrative but rarely metastasise.

Age incidence

- Approximately 10 years.
- No sex predilection.

Breed predisposition

- None.

Appearance

- Usually single, poorly circumscribed firm or fleshy masses 0.5–12 cm in diameter.

Diagnosis

- Biopsy.

Treatment

- Wide surgical excision.

LYMPHOCYTIC TUMOURS

LYMPHOMA

- May be:
  - ○ Non-epitheliotrophic – affecting dermal and subcutaneous tissue.
  - ○ Epitheliotrophic – lymphocytes manifest epitheliotrophism.

Non-epitheliotrophic lymphoma

Age incidence

- Usually greater than 10 years of age.
- No sex or breed predisposition.

Appearance

- Cutaneous manifestations:
  - ○ Usually generalised or multi-focal – rarely pruritic.
  - ○ Nodules present in almost all cases, firm, dermal or subcutaneous, often alopecic (Fig. 18.8).
  - ○ Exfoliative erythroderma an uncommon finding.
  - ○ Solitary lesion uncommon.
- Systemic involvement common, hypercalcaemia rare in the cat.

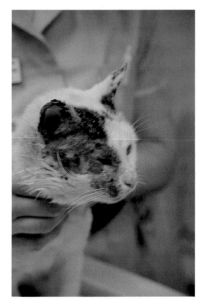

Fig. 18.8 Non-epitheliotrophic lymphoma showing alopecic nodules and plaques.

Diagnosis

- Fine needle aspirate of nodules.
- Impression smears of ulcers not always helpful – may reveal atypical lymphocytes.
- Biopsy – dermal and subcutaneous infiltration by malignant lymphocytes.

Treatment

- Poor prognosis – most cases progressive with development of more cutaneous lesions and metastasis to internal organs.
- Debatable whether treatment should be encouraged especially in FeLV positive animals. Recurrence rates are high.
- Treatment – poor response but therapy may give short-term remission.
  - Chemotherapy – combinations of prednisolone, cyclophosphamide, vincristine and cytosine arabinoside.
  - Surgical excision – solitary nodules.

Epitheliotrophic lymphoma

- An uncommon neoplasm of T lymphocytes.
- May be associated with FeLV.

Age incidence

- Greater than 9 years of age.
- No sex or breed predisposition.

Appearance

- Different clinical presentations can occur:
  - Exfoliative erythroderma often accompanied by alopecia (erythema with pruritus and scale).
  - Solitary or multiple erythematous plaques. Lesions pruritic leading to self-inflicted trauma and ulceration.
  - Solitary (occasionally multiple) intradermal nodules.

Diagnosis

- Fine needle aspirate of nodules and plaques.
- Impression smears of ulcers – Diff Quik stains reveal atypical lymphocytes.
- Biopsy – typical 'Pautrier' microabscesses.

Treatment.

- Poor prognosis – most cases progressive with development of more cutaneous lesions and metastasis to internal organs.
- Debatable whether treatment should be encouraged especially in FeLV positive animals. Recurrence rates are high.

- Treatment – poor response but therapy may give short-term remission.
  - ○ Chemotherapy – combinations of prednisolone, cyclophosphamide, vincristine and cytosine arabinoside.
  - ○ Surgical excision – solitary nodules.
  - ○ Retinoids – isotretinoin, etretinate.
  - ○ Other therapy which has been used includes topical nitrogen mustard, cyclosporin, omega-3 and omega-6 fatty acids, PEG–L-asparaginase – limited success rate seen with these therapies.

MELANOCYTIC NEOPLASMS

Melanocytoma

- Benign proliferation of melanocytes in the skin.

Age incidence

- Approximately 10 years.
- No sex predilection.

Breed predisposition

- None.

Appearance

- Usually solitary, well circumscribed alopecic firm brown or black nodules 0.5–4.0 cm in diameter.
- Site – head (especially pinna and nose) and neck.

Diagnosis

- Fine needle aspirate – presence of melanocytes.
- Biopsy – will identify as melanocytic neoplasm, but will not reliably differentiate melanocytoma from melanoma.

Treatment

- Radical surgical excision.

Melanoma

- Uncommon malignant proliferation of melanocytes in the skin.

Age incidence

- Approximately 10 years.
- Females predisposed.

Breed predisposition

- None.

Appearance

- Usually solitary, variable shape and colour usually brown or black, 0.5–4 cm in diameter, frequently ulcerated.
- Site – head (especially pinna, eyelid (Fig. 18.9) and lip), neck, back, tail and limbs.

Diagnosis

- As melanocytoma.

Treatment

- Radical surgical excision.

SECONDARY SKIN NEOPLASMS

- Secondary skin neoplasms occur by metastatic spread of primary neoplasms in other organs to the skin.
  - Metastatic bronchial carcinoma/squamous cell carcinoma of the lungs.
  - Thymoma/thoracic lymphoma.
  - Pancreatic paraneoplastic alopecia.

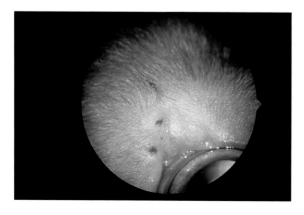

Fig. 18.9 Melanomas on the eyelid (picture courtesy of P. Boydell).

Metastatic bronchial carcinoma/squamous cell carcinoma of the lungs

- Asymptomatic thoracic lesions produce metastatic disease in the skin.

Age incidence
- Old cats.
- No sex predisposition.

Breed predisposition
- None.

Appearance
- Ulcerative, destructive paronychial lesions (Fig. 18.10).
- Always seen on multiple digits on multiple paws.
- Lesions may be pruritic.

Diagnosis
- Biopsy of lesions on digits.
- Thoracic X-rays.

Treatment
- Unsuccessful.

Thymoma

- Rare cutaneous lesions of erythroderma as a cutaneous manifestation of a thymoma.

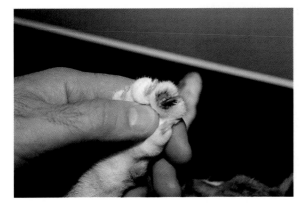

Fig. 18.10 Metastatic bronchial carcinoma producing destructive paronychial lesions.

Age incidence

- Adult to aged cats.
- No sex predisposition.

Breed predisposition

- None.

Appearance

- Non-pruritic scaling lesions initially leading to exfoliative erythroderma (Fig. 18.11) and alopecia with oozing erosions and ulcers.
- Brown waxy keratosebaceous debris accumulates between the toes and clawbeds.
- Site – lesions begin on the head, pinnae and neck, but rapidly generalise.

Diagnosis

- Biopsy of skin – erythema multiforme-like lesions.
- Thoracic X-rays.

Treatment

- Thymomas are generally benign and thus successful surgical excision of the thoracic mass has been shown to lead to resolution of the skin disease.

Pancreatic paraneoplastic alopecia

- See Chapter 8.

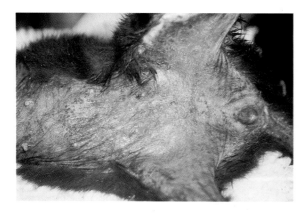

Fig. 18.11 Typical exfoliative erythroderma seen secondary to thymoma (picture courtesy of H. O'Dair).

NON-NEOPLASTIC TUMOURS

Cutaneous cysts

- Non-neoplastic, sac like structures with an epithelial lining.

Types of cyst

- Follicular cyst most common – often contain caseous yellow/brown material.
- Dermoid cyst – rare developmental abnormality.
- Apocrine sweat gland cysts – rare type of cyst in the cat caused by obstruction of sweat gland.
- Sebaceous gland cyst – very rare cyst derived from sebaceous gland.

Diagnosis and treatment

- Surgical removal – histopathology of cyst will indicate tissue of origin and therefore type.
- Benign neglect.
- Cyst should never be squeezed as this can incite a foreign body reaction if contents are lost into the dermis.

Nevi

- Uncommon developmental defect characterised by hyperplasia of one or more skin components.
- Those reported in the cat include:
  - Organoid nevi – hyperplasia of two or more skin components.
  - Apocrine sweat gland nevi.
  - Pancinian corpuscle nevi.

Cutaneous horn

- Uncommon cutaneous lesion in the cat.
- May originate from papillomas, basal cell tumours, squamous cell carcinomas, or actinic keratoses.

Age incidence

- None.
- No sex predisposition.

Breed predisposition

- None.

Appearance

- May be single or multiple.
- Firm horn-like projections up to 5 cm in length.
- Sites – multiple lesions on the footpads have been associated with FeLV infections, occasionally seen on the face.

Diagnosis

- Biopsy of skin – extensive compact hyperkeratosis; biopsies should always include the base of the horn.

Treatment

- Surgical excision.
- Observation without treatment.

Further Reading

Bonagura, J.D. (ed.) (1995) *Kirk's Current Veterinary Therapy XII*. W.B. Saunders, Philadelphia.

Bostock, D.E. and Owen, L.N. (1975) *Neoplasia in the Cat, Dog and Horse*. Yearbook Medical Publishers, Chicago.

Bush, B.M. (1991) *Interpretation of Laboratory Results for Small Animal Clinicians*. Blackwell Scientific, Oxford.

Carter, G.R. and Cole, J.R. (1990) *Diagnostics Procedures in veterinary bacteriology and Mycology V*. Academic Press, New York.

Carter, G.R. and Chengappa, M.M. (1991) *Essentials of Veterinary Bacteriology and Mycology IV*. Lea and Febiger, Philadephia.

Ettinger, S.J. (1989) *Textbook of Veterinary Internal Medicine III*. W.B. Saunders, Philadelphia.

Feldman, E.C. and Nelson, R.W. (1987) *Canine and Feline Endocrinology and Reproduction*. W.B. Saunders, Philadelphia.

Georgi, J. and Georgi, M. (1990) *Parasitology for Veterinarians*, 5th edn. W.B. Saunders, Philadelphia.

Goldschmidt, N.H. and Shofer, F. (1992) *Skin Tumours of the Dog and Cat*. Pergamon Press, New York.

Green, C.E. (1990) *Infectious Disease of the dog and cat*. W.B. Saunders, Philadelphia.

Griffin, C.A., Kwochka, K.W. and MacDonald, J.M. (eds) (1993) *Current Veterinary Dermatology*. Moseby Year Book, St Louis.

Gross, T.L., Ihrke, P.J. and Walder, E.J. (1992) *Veterinary Dermatopathology*. Moseby Year Book, St Louis.

Halliwell, R.E.W. and Gorman, N.T. (1989) *Veterinary Clinical Immunology*. W.B. Saunders, Philadelphia.

Holzworth, J. (1987) *Diseases of the Cat: Medicine and Surgery*. W.B. Saunders, Philadelphia.

Ihrke, P.J., Mason, I.S. and White, S.D. (eds) (1993) *Advances in Veterinary Dermatology*, Vol. 2. Pergamon Press, Oxford.

Kwochka, K.W., Willemse, T. and Tscharner, C. von (eds) (1998) *Advances in Veterinary Dermatology*, Vol. 3. Butterworth Heinemann, Oxford.

Lewis, L.D. and Morris, M.L. Jr (1984) *Small Animal Clinical Nutrition*, 2nd edn. Mark Morris Associates, Topeka.

Lewis, R.M. and Picut, C.A. (1989) *Veterinary Clinical Immunology*. Lea and Febiger, Philadelphia.

Moulton, J.E. (1990) *Tumours in Domestic Animals III*. University of California Press, Berkeley.

Reedy, L.M. and Miller, W.H. Jr. (1989) *Allergic Skin Diseases in Dogs and Cats*. W.B. Saunders, Philadelphia.

Stone, J. (1985) *Dermatology, Immunology and Allergy*. Moseby Year Book, St Louis.

Theilen, G.H. and Madewell, B.R. (1987) *Veterinary Cancer Medicine II*. Lea and Febiger, Philadelphia.

Thiers, B.H. and Dobson, R.L. (1986) *Pathogenesis of Skin Disease*. Churchill Livingstone, New York.

Tizard, I.R. (1992) *Veterinary Immunology: Introduction IV*. W.B. Saunders, Philadelphia.

Scott, D.W., Miller, W.H. and Griffin, C.E. (1995) *Muller and Kirk's Small Animal Dermatology*, 5th edn. W.B. Saunders, Philadelphia.

Tscharner, C. von and Halliwell, R.E.W. (eds) (1990) *Advances in Veterinary Dermatology*, Vol. 1. Ballière Tindall, London.

Withrow, S.J. and MacEwen, E.G. (1989) *Clinical Veterinary Oncology*. J.B. Lippincott, Philadelphia.

Yager, J.A. and Wilcox, B.P. (1994) *Colour Atlas and Text of Surgical Pathology of the Dog and Cat. Dermatopathology and Skin Tumours*. Wolfe, London.

Index